# PRACTICING WITHOUT "EVIDENCE"

FOR PRACTICING PEDIATRICIANS,
NEONATOLOGIST & JUNIOR DOCTORS

## Dr. ALOKE V.R

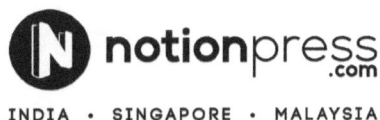

INDIA • SINGAPORE • MALAYSIA

**Notion Press Media Pvt Ltd**

No. 50, Chettiyar Agaram Main Road,
Vanagaram, Chennai, Tamil Nadu – 600 095

First Published by Notion Press 2021
Copyright © Dr. Aloke V.R 2021
All Rights Reserved.

ISBN 978-1-63904-670-6

This book has been published with all efforts taken to make the material error-free after the consent of the author. However, the author and the publisher do not assume and hereby disclaim any liability to any party for any loss, damage, or disruption caused by errors or omissions, whether such errors or omissions result from negligence, accident, or any other cause.

While every effort has been made to avoid any mistake or omission, this publication is being sold on the condition and understanding that neither the author nor the publishers or printers would be liable in any manner to any person by reason of any mistake or omission in this publication or for any action taken or omitted to be taken or advice rendered or accepted on the basis of this work. For any defect in printing or binding the publishers will be liable only to replace the defective copy by another copy of this work then available.

# Dedication

To my Patients for their selfless dedication and confidence shown towards me,

To my Teachers who taught me the basics and gave me a strong foundation,

To my Parents for the freedom and guidance given to live my dream,

To my Wife and children for their constant encouragement given,

To my Lord for placing me at the right place at right time.

**"CHANGE IS THE ONLY UNCHANGING REALITY IN THE UNIVERSE"**

# CONTENTS

*Preface*   9

1. Why is Immediate Survival from Paediatric In-hospital Cardiac Arrest (PIHCA) low? Is there an Inherent Fault in PALS Guidelines?   13

2. Tissue Circulation and Physiology during Shock and Normal – A Different Perspective (Oxygen-Glucose Dyad)   47

3. Which is the Main King Pin in Cellular Damage, Shock or Hypoxia?   56

4. CNS Microcirculation, Subtle Shock and Brain Damage   62

5. Microanalysis of Pediatric Cardiac Arrythmia during Sepsis-Shock Induced Cardiac Arrest   74

6. Is Subtle Shock the Hidden Monster in Brain Damage?   82

7. Does Tissue Level Hypoglycemia Always Accompany Shock? (Concept of Tissue Level Hypoglycemia)   95

8. Can Seizure be a Manifestation of Shock?   98

9. Referring a Sick Neonate – a Real Dilemma   101

10. Venous Blood Gas on Admission & Diluted Sodium Bicarbonate Helps to Quickly Stabilize Sick Babies on Admission to NICU   108

11. Abdominal Pain- Does Ultrasound Abdomen and Panic Always Warrened?   114

## Contents

12. NYLE Technique of Replacing Blocked PICC Line When Re-cannulation is Extremely Difficult ..... 123
13. Managing a Baby with Critical Serum Bilirubin of 28mg/dl (How to Tactically Avoid Exchange Transfusion without compromising the baby?) ..... 127
14. Apnea as a Manifestation of Early Shock ..... 134
15. Managing a Very Sick Term Baby Delivered Outside and Reaching you in a Very Bad State ..... 141
16. How can you Easily Treat Breath Holding Spells (BHS)? ..... 156
17. Managing a Gasping Baby Referred to you (Playing Gods Role) ..... 158
18. Speech Delay and Vitamin D Deficiency ..... 173
19. Early Features of Autism and Vitamin D Deficiency ..... 177
20. Development Delay or Lag and Vitamin D Deficiency ..... 180
21. An Overview of Mechanisms of Development Delay ..... 186
22. Pitfalls in the Management of Developmental Delay ..... 191
23. In-Utero Sepsis-Shock-Sequence (SSS) and Development Delay ..... 212
24. Is Eczema Always an "Allergic" Chronic Disease or a Treatable Disease? ..... 227
25. How to Handle the Complain of Loss of Appetite in a Child? ..... 233
26. Constipation: Is Symptomatic Treatment Enough, a Doctor's Dilemma ..... 239
27. How to Link Growth Failure with Chronic Asymptomatic and Symptomatic Throat Infections? ..... 246

| | | |
|---|---|---|
| 28. | Insight into Colonization, Reinfection and Incompletely Treated Primary Infection in a Child | 252 |
| 29. | Indian "Jugaad" Way of "No- Extra Cost" Safe Cooling for HIE | 266 |
| 30. | Is Incompletely Treated URTI the Main Cause of Community Spread and Disease Burden in the Community? | 270 |
| 31. | Is "Allergy" a Scapegoat Diagnosis? | 285 |
| 32. | Is There any Relationship Between Seizures and Vitamin D? | 291 |
| 33. | Clinically Noted Associations of Vitamin D Deficiency with Diseases and Mechanisms of Action of Vitamin D | 294 |
| 34. | Pitfalls in Seizure Management | 302 |
| 35. | A Passing Comment on Normal Distribution Curve (Gaussian Distribution) | 306 |
| 36. | Pitfalls Leading to Breastfeeding Failure | 309 |
| 37. | How to Prevent Antibiotic Misuses in Our Country? | 317 |
| 38. | Whole-Body Cooling in Resistant Neonatal Seizures as a Neuro Protective Strategy. | 321 |

*References*            *323*

# PREFACE

What is the need for another book when plenty of them are already available with the click of a button? This book is a compilation of experiences and observations of my career till date. A person's life is an amalgamation of experiences over the years and people write it down when it seems worth sharing. That is why people write autobiographies. My book is not an autobiography, it shares my experiences and observations over the years in Paediatrics and Neonatology. Some are not just observations but went beyond that to evolve into theories and have been useful in my clinical practice. Seeing its utility, I am compelled to write it down so that more and more patients would benefit and also needs to undergo greater scrutiny.

In today's world new observations and ideas need solid evidence for approval and appreciation. That is a good protective strategy against mismanagement towards patients. Proving all treatment strategies through studies is not possible in one's life time. We must understand that studies also have its own inherent limitations. When common sense can prove something to be worthy, is there a need for an elaborate study? May be needed depending on the subject.

This book is not a standard text, nor is a text describing treatment protocols. It is a compilation of observations made by me over 15 years of my clinical practice. I have made some clinically useful observations in the field of developmental delay, speech delay, children with early autistic features, theories regarding upper respiratory infections, constipation, abdominal pain, vomiting, sepsis and shock, seizures, wonders with judicious use of soda bicarbonate.

My most important observations are regarding PALS resuscitation guidelines, which according to me needs major restructuring. My aim is to dislodge everybody from their comfortable zones and stimulate intense discussions in this topic and arrive at a new normal.

Newer modalities of treatment definitely need stringent scrutiny through RCT's, meta-analysis etc. But don't discard a good observation of a good clinician from anywhere in the world. There is a clear divide between the practicing clinicians and academicians. The gap is widening with academicians asking for more and more evidence. Clinicians with their limited time and resources are tired of doing studies and publishing it is even more difficult. Clinicians should make their own platforms for bringing their view point.

Studies are beyond reach of vast majority of doctors who are working in an ordinary set up. But still, they observe a lot from their daily practice but are unable to prove it or convey to the larger audience. I am one such doctor, who unable to prove my experiences is writing a book to express my views. I wish this book will help individual patients to improve their quality of lives.

I encourage more and more practicing doctors with tons of observations to share their experience through books, because we are "forbidden" from journal publications.

My humble request is to critically analyse this book and subject it to studies and apply on patients wherever seems harmless, but don't criticise blindly for lack of evidence. My evidence are my patients. Remember my cover title Practicing without "Evidence".

Even if you have an idea, bringing it to the open is difficult. Finding a good publisher was a painstaking process but I think I made the right decision by choosing Notion Press publications. The reception

I received was unique and their platform is simply wonderful. I thank them whole heartedly and wishing them a brighter future.

**Dr. ALOKE V. R.**

**MD, DCH, DM (Neonatology)**

**Email: alokemybook@gmail.com**

## Chapter 1

# WHY IS IMMEDIATE SURVIVAL FROM PAEDIATRIC IN-HOSPITAL CARDIAC ARREST (PIHCA) LOW? IS THERE AN INHERENT FAULT IN PALS GUIDELINES?

From experience and from reading it was noticed that there is a wide difference in immediate survival between **Paediatric in-hospital cardiac arrest (PIHCA)** and **Neonatal in hospital cardiac arrest (NIHCA)**. Paediatric in-hospital survival from cardiac arrest is very low when compared to neonatal in-hospital cardiac arrest. Institutional and regional variations are there but generally speaking the PIHCA survival is low. On comparing and analysing the methods of resuscitation, there are difference in approaches between these two. This write up is to find out whether this difference in approach or some other factors are having any bearing on the survival. The paediatric in-hospital survival from cardiac arrest has improved significantly over the year in developed countries. This survival is still very low in developing countries. I am not going into the percentage statistics to prove PIHCA is low.

Even though neonatal period, infancy, childhood and adulthood are a continuum of one person's life, they are dealt differently when it comes to resuscitation. These subgroups are handled by different committees on resuscitation. Huge difference is seen between neonatal and other guidelines so also its survival.

Neonatal cardiac arrest is mainly due to a respiratory problem and heart is almost normal, so here arrythmia is less of a problem. But in adult cardiac arrest the heart is mainly the culprit and arrythmia is the main cause for arrest, mainly from myocardial infarction. In

Paediatric population, cardiac arrest usually results from one of the three following problems.

- Progressive respiratory distress and failure (the most common cause)
- Progressive shock (second most common)
- Sudden cardiac death from ventricular fibrillation (VF) or pulseless ventricular tachycardia (VT) (5-15% of all paediatric cardiac arrest cases)

In the following discussion cardiac arrest (CA) due to some special situations like congenital heart disease (CHD), CA due to pure arrhythmia (without any underlying diseases) are excluded. For convenience we will divide the resuscitation groups into three groups namely neonatal resuscitation group (≤ 28 days), infant and paediatric group (>28 days to 18 years) and the adult group. Outside hospital cardiac arrest is not discussed here. Let us compare between these groups.

**Table: 1**  Comparison of Resuscitation between groups

| Parameters | Neonatal (≤ 28days) (NALS-7$^{th}$ ed) | Infant & children (PALS-2015) | Adult (ACLS-2015) |
|---|---|---|---|
| Primary problem | Mainly respiratory | Mostly respiratory | Majority cardiac |
| When will you resuscitate? | Apnoea /gasping / HR<100 | Apnoea / gasping / HR <60 | Apnoea / gasping / no pulse |
| Initial approach | Bag & mask (B&G) | B & M | B & M |

| Parameters | Neonatal (≤ 28days) (NALS-7th ed) | Infant & children (PALS-2015) | Adult (ACLS-2015) |
|---|---|---|---|
| CPR cycle – Breath rate | 40-60 bpm (isolated IPPV)<br><br>30/ min (combined with chest compression) | 8 or 16 breaths /min<br><br>(depending on number of rescuers) | 8 breaths / min |
| CPR cycle – Chest compression rate | 90 /min | 100-120/ min | 100-120/min |
| CPR Compression: Breath ratio | 90:30 (3:1) (120 events/min) | 15:2 | 30:2 |
| Respiratory rate | Adequate respiratory rate for age | Respiratory rate low, below physiological | Respiratory rate low, but adequate for age |
| Intubation | Early and time bound (within 1-1/2 mins) | No time line and late | No time line |
| In hospital CA survival rates | Good | Low | Low |

For those who are working both in Neonatal and Paediatric intensive care units it is a known fact that there is a higher rate of survival after Neonatal cardiac arrest when compared to a cardiac arrest in paediatric intensive care. (by cardiac arrest it does not always means stoppage of heart, it also includes situations where if reasonable actions are not taken heart will stop in immediate future). When you are resuscitating a newborn you can be reasonably sure that you can save the child, but that is not the case with paediatric resuscitation, there is more chance of losing the baby. Our experience shows that almost >90 % of newborn CA cases can be revived without much difficulty unless it is a bad terminal case. But that is not the case with paediatric CA cases where survival rates are in the range of < 25%. This is a serious difference as physiology remains the same only the age is different. From curiosity I dug deeper into the intricate mechanisms leading to death during cardiac arrest. I found some clues which can be of help in improving the outcome.

**For explaining my point let us take a case scenario of death in an eight-month-old child with severe pneumonia, sepsis and shock.** As the child's infection progresses there are changes happening in different parameters in the body. There is progressive hypoxia, gradual build-up of carbon dioxide, metabolic acidosis, shock, increasing base deficit, electrolyte changes, seizures, huge release of immune mediators, counter regulatory hormone release, accumulation of excitatory neurotransmitters, depletion of ATP in the brain, cardiac muscles and other tissues etc.

**Table: 2** Child's progressive deterioration through sequence 1 to 5

| Parameters | Sequence-1 | Sequence-2 | Sequence-3 | Sequence-4 | Sequence-5 |
|---|---|---|---|---|---|
| Time | 0 hrs | 1 hr | 2 hr | 3 hr | 3.10 hr |
| pH | **7.325** | **7.29** | **7.18** | **7.07** | **6.8** |
| $PaCO_2$ | 32 | 26 | 47 | 64 | 75 |
| $PaO_2$ | 60 | 50 | 40 | 39 | 25 |
| $HCO_3$ | 16 | 11 | 8 | 6 | 4 |
| BE | -7 | -10 | -16 | -19 | -22 |
| $SPO_2$ | 97 | 92 | 86 | 76 | 66 |
| Na | 135 | 130 | 129 | 123 | 122 |
| K | 4.5 | 5.2 | 5.8 | 6.4 | 6.8 |

| Parameters | Sequence-1 | Sequence-2 | Sequence-3 | Sequence-4 | Sequence-5 |
|---|---|---|---|---|---|
| *iCa++ | Normal | Low normal | Low | Low | Low |
| Shock | Early shock | Shock | Advance shock | Circulatory collapse | Circulatory collapse |
| Peripheral circulation | CRT prolonged | CRT prolonged | CRT prolonged | CRT prolonged | CRT prolonged |
| BP | Normal / high | Normal /Low | Low BP | Hypotension | Hypotension |
| Respiration | Tachypnoea | Tachypnoea & Resp. distress | Tachypnoea & Resp. distress | Gasping | Apnoea |
| Heart Rate | Tachycardia develops | Tachycardia | tachycardia | **Bradycardia** | Arrest |
| Vital organ – Brain | Preserved (agitated) | Compromised (agitated, seizures) | Drowsy (seizures) | Drowsy | Stupor |

| Parameters | Sequence-1 | Sequence-2 | Sequence-3 | Sequence-4 | Sequence-5 |
|---|---|---|---|---|---|
| Vital organ – Heart | Preserved | Compromised | Compromised | Chance for arrhythmia | Arrest |
| Vital organ – Kidney | Preserved | Compromised | compromised | Kidney shutdown | Non functional |
| Comments | Mild $CO_2$ wash out / metabolic acidosis developing | Metabolic acidosis with compensatory resp. alkalosis / hypotension developing | Metabolic + resp. acidosis. Decompensated shock / possibility of arrythmia increases | Resp. acidosis. Decompensated shock / arrhythmia. Any time arrest. Heart start to fail | Resp. arrest / cardiac arrest |

* usually, metabolic acidosis produces increase in ionic Ca++, but most critical babies have low ionic ca++

This child progressively goes into cardiac arrest. Either child goes into gradual bradycardia and arrest or directly goes into arrhythmia and arrest. Let us analyse the blood parameters on the way to arrest.

**Table: 3**  Pre-Arrest Parameters and Observations

| Pre arrest Parameters | | Observations | |
|---|---|---|---|
| pH | 6.8 | Acidosis can lead to death (both respiratory & metabolic), cellular enzymatic functions are extremely suppressed, severe myocardial depression occurs. | Respiratory alkalosis rarely cause death but metabolic alkalosis can lead to death, usually during poisoning |
| $PaCO_2$ | 75 | Terminal stages $PaCO_2$ raises | Respiratory arrest and $PaCO_2$ build up |
| $PaO_2$ | 25 | Hypoxia causes death | Fetus survives in extreme low $PaO_2$ conditions with no problem/ low $PaO_2$ causes body to shift into anaerobic metabolism, even though inefficient there is an available alternative. |
| $HCO_3$ | 4 | A buffer | Gets exhausted / regeneration of $HCO_3$ is by kidney and is a slow process, highly inefficient during poor circulation, shock & cardiac arrest conditions. |
| BE | -22 | Gives an idea about the base deficit body is facing | $HCO_3$ was used up to neutralize H+ ions produced from lactic acid and other sources |

| Pre arrest Parameters | | Observations | |
|---|---|---|---|
| SPO2 | 66 | It represents the % of Hb molecules which are saturated. Hypoxia – cells shifted to anaerobic metabolism (highly inefficient) | 19 times less efficient compared to aerobic metabolism (aerobic: anaerobic, 36 ATP: 2 ATP). So, 19 times more glucose required to maintain ATP status co. |
| Na (↓) | 122 | Hyponatremia – due to multiple mechanisms, also due to imbalanced shifting of Na in and out of cells | Chance of seizure increases but not much effect on cardiac muscles (?) Na-K ATPase malfunction due to ATP deficiency |
| K (↑) | 6.8 | Hyperkalaemia can cause death through arrhythmia (sustained depolarization) & from poor cardiac muscle contractility. (K+ shifts out of cells during metabolic acidosis in exchange for H+ ions) | Chances of cardiac arrest high. K+ Rapidly raises after arrest. (multiple mechanisms) Na-K ATPase malfunction due to ATP deficiency, from cell lysis etc. |
| iCa++ (↓) | Low iCa++ | Role in cardiac arrhythmia (low Ca2+ and high K+ can exaggerate chance for arrythmia) | Cardiac contraction becomes weak |

| Pre arrest Parameters | | Observations | |
|---|---|---|---|
| Glucose | Usually, high due to stress | Counter regulatory hormones keep glucose very high during crisis | Since anaerobic metabolism is highly inefficient consumption of glucose may be high, blood glucose may be high but inside the cell it may be low because of increased consumption, so added hypoglycaemia produces very bad outcome. |

Normally all cells are in a polarised state with outside of cells positively charged and inside of the cells negatively charged. This polarity is maintained in the cell membrane by the action of Na-K ATPase activity and that requires continuous supply of ATP (energy currency of cell). Whenever this supply is disrupted, cellular function starts to deteriorate and malfunction (in brain it manifests as seizures, alteration in sensorium, in the heart as arrhythmia, poor cardiac contractility etc). This is the case in every cell in the body.

Any change in blood pH or ATP supply disruption affects the functioning of the Na-K ATPase and in turn effects the cell membrane polarity. This polarity represents the vitality of the cell. Na-K ATPase enzyme is highly pH sensitive enzyme.

A deteriorating septic baby invariably shows moderate to severe acidosis (metabolic and or respiratory acidosis). Never seen a baby deteriorating with a normal ABG, unless due to a pure arrhythmia. Why is that? **Baby's deterioration is highly linked with blood pH changes rather than to its oxygenation.**

During shock when the blood pH drops (↑H+) there is shifting of H+ ions from blood to the inside of cells and in exchange K+ shifts out of the cells resulting in hyperkalaemia (this is not directly as it seems, through H-K ATPase & Na-K ATPase). Normally there is a dynamic balance between Na+ movement into and out of cell and K+ movement out of the cell through the action of Na-K ATPase. When Na-K ATPase falters due to energy deficiency Na+ gets trapped inside the cell resulting in hyponatremia outside the cell and hypernatremia inside the cell. This produces water retention inside the cell resulting in cellular oedema. In short, this cell membrane pump failure can result in cellular functional failure and cell death and groups of cell death result in necrosis of a tissue and which ultimately leads to death of that person.

ATP production is an end result of a multitude of enzymatic reactions, participation of several cellular organelles (mitochondria, endoplasmic reticulum, cytoplasmic enzymes etc.). All these enzymatic activities are pH dependent and function maximally at a particular pH. Any deviation from that pH will only decrease its activity. For ATP production, a continuous supply of glucose and oxygen are required. When there is oxygen deficiency, cells shift to anaerobic metabolism which is an inefficient method of ATP production (efficiency 18 times less, 36 ATP Vs 2 ATP production). Anaerobic metabolism produces lactic acid as its end product. Lactic acidosis in the blood is an indirect indication of anaerobic metabolism in the body. To neutralise this acid buffering systems come into play and bicarbonate ions plays a major role in neutralizing these acids. At extremes of acidosis, buffering systems fails and blood pH falls rapidly. For optimal cellular function blood pH should be kept between 7.35 and 7.45, and any pH below 7.25 results in rapid cellular functional deterioration.

## What is brain death or for that matter death?

- Is death the loss of viability of some unknown vital centres in brain?

- Or death occurs when most part of the brain becomes unviable (isoelectric EEG)
- Or death occurs when inner core part of brain becomes unviable – Basal ganglia, Thalamus, Hypothalamus, Brain stem etc. (dilated fixed pupil is a good sign of brain death).

Brain death is a complex question still not satisfactorily answered. What is the most important parameter leading to cell death, is it **Blood pH deviation, Hypoxia, tissue level hypoglycaemia, hypercarbia, or hyperkalaemia?**

A very sick septic child may be able to maintain life (maintain blood pH) for some time and then he/she trips and fall to death, paralleling with fall of blood pH. During that process pH nose dives and falls below 7.0, $PCO_2$ raises, hyperkalaemia and hypocalcaemia worsens and oxygenation falls to low levels and baby goes into apnoea, bradycardia and cardiac arrest or child directly goes into arrythmia and cardiac arrest. This is the common pathway leading to most deaths. Blood pH fall is the result of metabolic and or respiratory acidosis. During the initial stages of sepsis, metabolic acidosis is the sole cause of acidosis and later on when compensatory mechanisms fail respiratory acidosis sets in both of which nose dives blood pH, unless the primary cause is purely respiratory without sepsis. Fall in blood pH drives all cellular function haywire and death at cellular level ensures. You can survive with a blood PaCO2 >80 or 100, provided blood pH is maintained above 7.1 or 7.2 by buffering systems. Similarly, you can survive with severe metabolic acidosis with a bicarbonate value of 2 or 4 provided blood pH is kept above 7.1 or 7.2. But you cannot survive for long with a blood pH less than 7 with PCO2 or HCO3 in the near normal range. It is obvious that major determinant of cell survival is blood pH and pH alterations derails all cellular function and death ensures. So, it is obvious that **pH abnormality is affecting the cellular function the most** and all enzymatic functions are pH dependent and it goes haywire when it is abnormal. There are centres in the brain which tightly controls the blood pH in a narrow range. Multiple organs in the body (kidneys, lungs, blood buffering systems, chemoreceptors at multiple locations) are synchronizing with each other and coordinating to defend the blood pH in the normal range.

To defend any immediate blood pH changes body brings in buffering systems to its defence. (long-term corrections are through kidneys). When this defence mechanisms gets exhausted some external interventions have to come to its rescue to correct blood pH otherwise cellular death ensures. Actually, the ultimate aim of resuscitation should be to provide oxygenation and maintain circulation and also to defend near normal blood pH. In the current resuscitation guidelines blood pH maintenance is not a priority. If blood pH maintenance is a priority, then you have to take care of carbon dioxide washout, because it is the only immediately available compensation for metabolic acidosis. For that you have to keep a reasonably good respiratory rate and it should be efficient also. But current PALS guidelines only emphasis on **oxygenation and circulation** and no importance is given for the maintenance of normal blood pH. **Blood pH maintenance must be the ultimate goal in resuscitation.** If you try to defend blood pH you will have to take care of circulation and carbon dioxide washout. If you don't maintain circulation metabolic acidosis worsens. If you don't maintain carbon dioxide washout respiratory acidosis sets in and brings downs blood pH, the drop in blood pH will be very fast as both metabolic and respiratory acidosis acts in cohesion (same direction). Moreover, during resuscitation, we should be assisting the depleted buffering systems ($HCO_3$ buffering) because that helps in bringing blood pH to normal range. But current PALS guideline is not at all directed towards these things because of the misguided priority of only circulation and oxygenation. **During any crisis, our body is trying**

**to defend the blood pH, we need to only assist this.** If you are making carbon dioxide washout to maintain blood pH a priority then intubating the child becomes mandatory. This is the real crux of the problem, our training of undergraduate and graduates in intubation needs to be augmented and I will come to this part of discussion later.

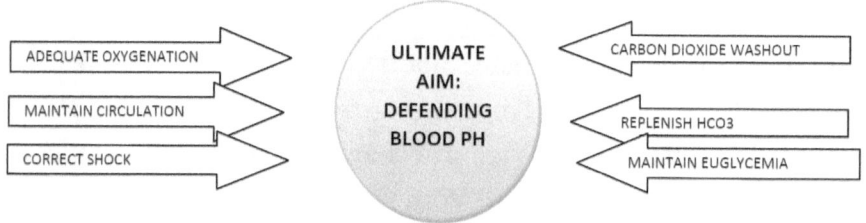

**Figure: 1** Defending blood pH

**Table: 4** Comparison of current PALS priority and suggested PALS priority

| Parameters | Current PALS priority | Suggested PALS priority |
|---|---|---|
| Circulation | Yes | Yes |
| Oxygenation | Yes | Yes |
| Blood pH maintenance | Not a priority | Make a priority |
| Carbon dioxide washout to maintain blood pH | Not a priority | Should be priority and consider early intubation & fast respiratory rate |
| Augmenting $HCO_3$ buffering capacity of blood | Not a priority | Should be priority and consider IV $HCO_3^-$ |
| Early intubation | Not a priority | Should be a priority |

During metabolic acidosis, hyperkalaemia develops and hyperkalaemia depresses heart and produces bradycardia and at any time it can cause arrythmia and sudden arrest. During the terminal 5 to 10 minutes preceding death the hyperkalaemia can rapidly peak following an inverse relationship with metabolic acidosis, at this point measurement of both metabolic acidosis and hyperkalaemia are difficult and not accurate. To compound the worsening condition in a critically ill child hypocalcaemia also creeps in. Calcium was supposed to counter the action of hyperkalaemia on heart but the opposite is happening that is hypocalcemia. All adds up to the severe myocardial depressant effect ending in myocardial failure and cardiac arrest. PALS guidelines in not giving any importance to these worsening parameters.

## CONCEPT OF "RESUSCITATION BLIND SPOT"

This is a period during resuscitation in which it is not possible to measure reliably any of the important blood parameters. It is a period during which panic button is pressed when child goes into bradycardia and arrest. This period includes immediate pre-arrest and arrest period during resuscitation. During resuscitation blind spot so many factors change rapidly, but we will not be able take measurements reliably because of our priority towards resuscitation and difficulty in extracting blood during that time. We have to assume things during this juncture and have to take appropriate decisions. Only in experimentally created animal studies or in patients with an arterial line we can get exact values. In majority of patients in a suboptimal set up this is a rarity. Let us see the blood parameters and they are, blood pH, $PCO_2$, $HCO_3$, $H+$, $K+$, $Ca^+$, $PO_2$, and $SPO_2$. Blood parameters like pH, $K^+$, $Ca^+$, $PCO_2$ values change dramatically in that panic and need to take decisions based on assumptions in majority of cases.

**Table: 5**  Parameter Changes During Resuscitation Blind Spot

| Parameters | Changes | Good or Bad | Effects |
|---|---|---|---|
| Blood pH | ↓ | Bad | All cellular functions deteriorate |
| $HCO_3^-$ | ↓ | Bad | Depletion of buffering system |
| $PO_2$ | ↓ | Bad | Hypoxic cellular damage |
| $Ca^{++}$ | ↓ | Bad | Cardiac depression |
| $Na^+$ | ↓ | Bad | Prone for seizures |
| $PCO_2$ | ↑ | Bad | Respiratory acidosis |
| $K^+$ | ↑ | Bad | Cardiac arrythmia & cardiac arrest |
| BE | ↓ | Bad | Shows depleted buffering system |
| $H^+$ | ↑ | Bad | Acidosis |
| ATP | ↓ | Bad | Energy depletion in cells |
| Excitatory amino acid accumulation | ↑ | Bad | Produce seizures |

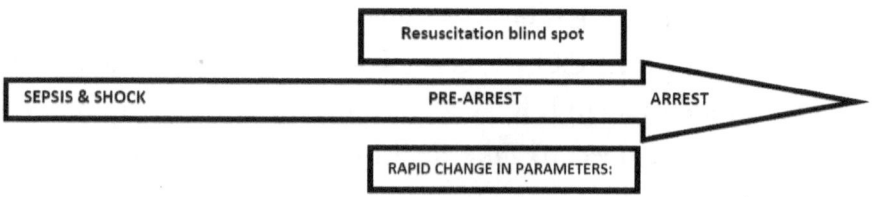

**Figure: 2**  Resuscitation blind spot

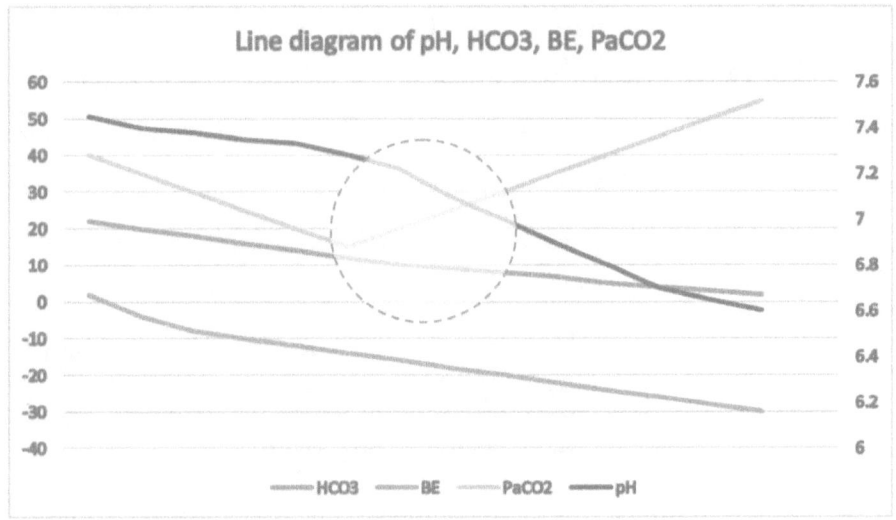

**Figure: 3**   Changes during Resuscitation Blind Spot

Let us discuss the blood parameters just before cardiac arrest with an example. Blood parameters just before cardiac arrest in a child with sepsis, shock and pneumonia:

**ABG: PH: 6.9, BE: -22, K⁺: 6.4,** *PaCO$_2$: 75, PaO$_2$: 25, HCO$_3$: 4, iCa⁺: 1.01* (in bold – indirect parameters, which cannot be directly controlled) (in italics – directly controllable variables) (iCa⁺ = ionized calcium).

---

Brain damage due to shock ∞ Duration and severity of shock

---

The above are the blood parameters just before the cardiac arrest. Some are direct parameters (PaCO$_2$, PaO$_2$, HCO$_3$, iCa⁺) which can be corrected directly and others are indirect parameters (pH, BE, K⁺) which can be influenced directly. Actions which have to be done to save the child are,

1. Increase oxygenation to 100% (everybody will be giving 100% oxygen at this point)
2. We have to defend blood pH at any cost. This can be achieved by doing the following,
   a) By forcing carbon dioxide washout (as respiratory compensation)
   b) By giving IV soda bicarbonate (augment exhausted buffering capacity of blood)
   c) By better control of shock and sepsis
3. Washing out of carbon dioxide as a compensatory mechanism to bring back blood pH to near normal.
4. Counter measures to correct hyperkalaemia
5. Administration of soda bicarbonate to bring back blood pH to near normal. This action also causes decrease of hyperkalaemia, which is the real culprit in arrythmia and cardiac arrest (see subsequent chapters).
6. Administration of IV Calcium to counter the effects of hyperkalaemia and to augment the contractility of heart resulting in improved circulation.

Here it is obvious that to bring back pH to near normal levels either carbon dioxide has to be removed or we have to give IV soda bicarbonate as an alkalinising agent or do both. Usually, this alkalinisation is done by kidneys through a rather slow process, so not useful in acute emergencies like cardiac arrest. For washing out carbon dioxide we have to intubate and ventilate the child and give breaths at a higher rate. These two are not at all considered in the PALS guidelines. Don't give soda bicarbonate without securing the airway as this can worsens respiratory acidosis. Then intubation becomes compulsory rather than optional. You have to counter hyperkalaemia as hyperkalaemia seems to be the ultimate cause of cardiac arrest. Heart either enters into arrythmia or hearts stops in diastole due to extreme hyperkalaemia and hypocalcaemia. There is a terminal spike in the hyperkalaemia which is unmeasurable (during the resuscitation blind spot) and it keeps on increasing as time passes by because of increasing acidosis (respiratory and metabolic). This increase in acidosis cannot be countered by current guidelines (low respiratory rate, delayed intubation, and absence of soda bicarbonate infusion), this may be the reason for the increased mortality seen in paediatric resuscitation.

The carbon dioxide washout is not possible with the current system of **American Heart Association (AHA) recommended infant & child resuscitation guidelines** (PALS-2015) of 30:2 or 15:2 cardiac massage to breathe ratio. (using an Ambu bag). **The present PALS guidelines have given importance only to oxygenation and circulation and not to $CO_2$ washout or blood pH maintenance.** It is not possible to wash out carbon dioxide (as a counter to severe metabolic acidosis) without intubation. So, like in neonatal resuscitation we have to intubate early and the breath rates has to be increased substantially. This produces $CO_2$ washout and improves pH temporarily and helps in the revival of cardiac function. Through this process we are buying time for the correction of primary cause (sepsis, shock and acidosis). Moreover, there are no measures to counter **hyperkalaemia**, an old potassium value may not be the real K+ value nearing arrest ("resuscitation blind spot"), as potassium has a narrow safe zone and it increases rapidly with metabolic acidosis. As the baby becomes more critical there is development of hypocalcaemia, which worsens hyperkalaemia induced cardiac toxicity. Calcium is the one which counters actions of hyperkalaemia. There is no recommendation for IV calcium gluconate during paediatric resuscitation.

Current resuscitation stresses mainly on restoration of blood supply to heart through coronaries. This blood supply is mainly aimed at restoration of oxygen supply. My argument is just restoration of blood supply to heart without improving the grossly abnormal blood pH (with associated hyperkalaemia) will not revive heart function. Heart is failing because all the cellular functions are haywire due to enzymatic shutdown (all are pH dependent) and energy (ATP) deficiency. Heart is also highly arrhythmia prone when there is hyperkalaemia, cell membrane instability (due to Na-K ATPase malfunction) and when blood pH is abnormal.

The other method to improve blood pH is administration of soda bicarbonate (this is highly controversial due to "unknown" reasons). This rapidly corrects acidosis and bring pH to above 7. Soda bicarbonate administration is not possible without securing an airway, so intubation is a must during resuscitation. Administration of soda bicarbonate is a method to buy time until the primary cause that caused all these problems are corrected.

a) **Respiratory acidosis:** ------ Corrected through carbon dioxide washout: intubate and increase respiratory rate

b) **Metabolic acidosis:** ----- Correction by kidneys by retaining $HCO_3$ (not efficient during cardiac arrest). Alternative method is to give IV soda bicarbonate.

c) **Correction of hyperkalaemia:** direct correction of hyperkalaemia is not possible during arrest or during pre-arrest condition, the available options are to correct metabolic acidosis (IV soda bicarbonate) which in turn corrects hyperkalaemia. Another way is to counter the effects of hyperkalaemia is by administering IV calcium gluconate.

d) **Correction of hypocalcaemia or counter the actions of hyperkalaemia:** administer IV calcium during pre-arrest or during arrest to counter effects of hyperkalaemia or to prevent hypocalcaemia. Exact measurement of potassium values and calcium are nearly impossible during these acute conditions ("resuscitation blind spot").

In short through the above **four actions,** we can revive person from arrest. (You have only 3-5 minutes to do everything before cardiac arrest brings complete brain death).

- Respiratory acidosis correction through Carbon dioxide washout.
    - Intubate early
    - Use higher ventilatory rate
- Metabolic acidosis correction through
    - Intubate early and ventilate with higher rate (respiratory compensation to counter metabolic acidosis)
    - Administer diluted IV soda bicarbonate
- Counter effects of hyperkalaemia
    - IV Calcium
- Correct hypocalcaemia
    - IV Calcium

1. **Immediate intubation and ventilation with higher ventilation rate.**

Our usual ventilation rate of 30:2 for adults and 15:2 for children will not revive the patient if the cardiac arrest involves metabolic acidosis and or respiratory acidosis. Intubate and increase respiratory rates to 30-40 will help in washing out the excess carbon dioxide and helps in improving pH to above 7.2. Ventilation by using Bag & Mask is inefficient in washing our carbon dioxide but may be sufficient for oxygenation. Once pH is above 7.25, we can decrease the respiratory rates to normal physiologic levels based on ABG values. (select the ventilation rate you would have set for a person on ventilator with this amount of sickness). A more than higher ventilation rate (over ventilation) at this time is not going to harm the child. Simultaneously you have to correct the primary cause of sepsis and shock aggressively (higher antibiotics and inotropes) otherwise the cardiac arrest will revisit the child in a not-so-distant future.

Neonatal resuscitation is having higher success rate because of early intubation (within 1-1/2 minutes of non-improvement) and higher ventilation rates of 30-40 /minute and also because of the relative resistance of heart to arrythmia. This resistance may be because of the higher tolerance of neonatal heart towards hyperkalaemia.

2. **Correct metabolic acidosis through soda bicarbonate administration (taking over the kidney function of $HCO_3^-$ re-absorption).**

By giving soda bicarbonate as IV we can rapidly correct the pH, this can by-pass the slow $HCO_3^-$ reabsorption through renal tubules. This action (pH) improves cellular enzymatic functions and helps in rapidly restoring ATPs and also helps in bringing down hyperkalaemia. ATP deficiency and cell membrane pump failure are the root cause of all cell death. Immediate aim should be to bring pH values to above 7 and then to >7.25. With this pH the cellular function including that of cardiac muscles improves. Cardiac contraction improves once hyperkalaemia is corrected and cardiac muscle becomes less prone for arrythmia. All events are part of a chain reaction started with shock and metabolic acidosis and we have to reverse it one by one as quickly as possible.

3. **Correction of hyperkalaemia:** direct correction of hyperkalaemia is not possible during arrest or during pre-arrest conditions, the available options are to correct metabolic acidosis which in turn corrects hyperkalaemia. Another way to counter the effects of hyperkalaemia is through the administration of IV calcium. The bad role of hyperkalaemia in the events is never recognized before, so also the role of hypocalcaemia.

4. **Correction of hypocalcaemia or counter actions of hyperkalaemia:** Studies have shown that hypocalcaemia invariably accompanies sick conditions. Administer IV calcium during pre-arrest or during arrest to counter effects of hyperkalaemia and to counter hypocalcaemia. Exact measurement of potassium values and calcium values are nearly impossible during these acute conditions ("resuscitation blind spot", fig. 2 & 3).

During the "resuscitation blind spot" three events happen rapidly which usually escapes detection and so are not highlighted much. First event is the respiratory compensation failure (i.e. Development of respiratory acidosis) and raise of $PCO_2$ after which blood pH nose dives. This nose-diving blood pH elevates blood potassium level which is the second event happening, which is also difficult to measure. This raising potassium causes arrythmia and myocardial depression and arrest. The third event happening silently is the hypocalcaemia. The calcium is supposed to counter the hyperkalaemia but the opposite (hypocalcaemia) is happening. Usually, hypercalcaemia should accompany acidosis but in most sick babies it is the reverse happening because of multitude of cellular mechanisms.

**Major resuscitation blind spot events:**

- Failure of respiratory compensation and development of respiratory acidosis
- Rapid pH drop (acidosis)

- Rapid elevation of potassium levels
- Hypocalcaemia

**Table: 6** Different Emergency calls from an ICU nurse (Pre-arrest calls)

| Pre arrest call from a nurse on duty | Arrest condition | How to revive this child | Basic minimum needed to revive the condition |
|---|---|---|---|
| Saturation falling | No heart rate<br><br>No respiration<br><br>No saturation<br><br>Becomes unresponsive | Restore at least the minimum the baby was getting at the pre arrest condition<br><br>First pull back to the pre arrest condition<br><br>Restore respiration 30-40 /min<br><br>HR of 120/min<br>$SPO_2$ of 90 | Give ventilation & oxygen (intubation and ventilation is the best way)<br><br>External Cardiac Massage (ECM)<br><br>Drugs |
| Child goes into bradycardia | | | |
| Apnoea / irregular resp. / gasping | | | |
| Seizures and stiffening | | | |
| Child become limp and pale | | | |
| **Heart was pushed into arrest due to some unknown cause – we have to find the cause and correct it, mostly it is sepsis, shock, with or without arrythmia.** ||||

Here are some basic questions and trying to find some answers.

### 1. What is the ultimate aim of Paediatric resuscitation or for that matter any resuscitation?

Clinical death by definition is no heart rate, no respiration, no signs of life and dilated fixed pupils. For death to happen heart's pumping has to stop and all energy supply lines for vital organs has to stop. If heart stops completely for 3-5 minutes brain death will follow. So, first and foremost thing in resuscitation is restoration of activity of heart to normal, temporary functional restoration is external cardiac massage. We have to reverse the factors leading to cardiac arrest. The factors leading to cardiac arrest are,

- **Shock and acidosis (metabolic & respiratory) and its downward spiral.**
- **Hyperkalaemia and hypocalcaemia**
- **Arrythmia induced cardiac arrest** (acidosis, hyperkalaemia and hypocalcaemia induced)

a) **Shock and acidosis (metabolic & respiratory) and its downward spiral.**

Shock or poor blood supply leads to lack of oxygen and glucose supply to tissues and accumulation of $CO_2$. Shock also produces metabolic acidosis which also supresses cardiac function. In the later stages respiratory acidosis sets in. This $CO_2$ accumulation occurs when the body is not able to transport back carbon dioxide produced in the body due to shock (poor circulation due to poor cardiac function). In acute emergency oxygenation to heart is more important. So, try to improve oxygenation through bag and mask with 100% oxygen along with a low IPPV rate. Low IPPR rate is sufficient when oxygenation is the only concern. Action of shock on cardiac muscle is a type of vicious cycle, shock leading to poor blood supply to heart and which further deteriorates heart function and this again worsens shock. Another thing happening is blood pH drop, which in turn suppresses all cellular functions including that of myocardium. To counter metabolic acidosis option of carbon dioxide washout to bring pH to near normal was never considered till now. For most cases this slow IPPV with bag and mask technique worked. It may not work when blood pH is very low (pH below 7.1-7.0) or when accompanied by respiratory acidosis. Body's immediate compensation for metabolic acidosis is carbon dioxide washout, when this washout mechanism fails and respiratory acidosis sets in blood pH drops precipitously and monitoring this rapid fall in pH is very difficult ("resuscitation blind spot"). When the blood pH is very low like for example pH: 6.8 – 7.1 range the myocardium is really depressed and a vicious cycle sets in towards cardiac arrest. Here a quick intubation with higher IPPV rate would improve the blood pH and also the myocardial function. No amount of resuscitation with a slow IPPV (as recommended by PALS guidelines) with Bag & mask or after intubation is going to improve blood pH. As long as a we are not considering improvement in the blood pH (acidosis) we are not forced to change our resuscitation guidelines. For blood pH to improve, there should be carbon dioxide washout, for that early intubation is a necessity. After intubation we can give IV soda bicarbonate to improve the blood pH faster. **Due to lack of early intubation and higher resuscitation rate the use of soda bicarbonate to improve blood pH has been thrown into the back burner.** ABG taken at the time of severe shock or arrest may not reflect the actual cellular picture because of shock. That means because of shock the accumulated H+ ions may not be yet carried to the main circulation. So, each cell (myocardium) may be in more acidosis than shown by an ABG. That is why when you start correcting shock all acid ions flood the system later. If the myocardium is very much suppressed and goes into cardiac arrest all the events near the myocardial cells reaches exponential proportion and becomes non-measurable. The things happening are hyper acidosis, hyperkalaemia, hypocalcaemia, hypoxemia, local tissue hypoglycaemia (from over utilization and absent supply)

**Table: 7** Effects of Various Factors on Myocardium and Corrective Measures

| Shock | Cardiac muscle cell | Corrective measure |
|---|---|---|
| Hypoxemia | Shift towards anaerobic metabolism | 100 % $O_2$ |
| Accumulation of $CO_2$ | Respiratory acidosis develops, any acidosis supresses cellular function | Intubation and faster IPPR |
| Accumulation of lactate | pH falls, acidosis, cellular function deteriorates | IV $NaHCO_3$ |
| Low $HCO_3$ | Buffering capacity drops | IV $NaHCO_3$ |
| Hyperkalaemia | Depresses myocardium, induces arrythmia | IV calcium Correct acidosis IV $NaHCO_3$ Faster IPPR (metabolic and respiratory) |
| Hypocalcaemia | Cardiac depressant effect, worsens shock  Exaggerate effects of hyperkalaemia on myocardium | IV calcium |
| High base deficit | Shows exhausted buffering capacity | IV $NaHCO_3$ |
| Bradycardia / Arrest | Shock & Vicious cycle sets in | ECM + adrenaline |

| Shock | Cardiac muscle cell | Corrective measure |
|---|---|---|
| Very low pH (severe metabolic and or resp. acidosis) | Suppresses all cellular function including cardiac | IV $NaHCO_3$ + $CO_2$ washout through faster IPPR (intubation) |
| Apnoea | Hypoxia and accumulation of $CO_2$ | Intubation & IPPR |

### b) Hyperkalaemia and hypocalcaemia (detail discussion in separate chapter)

These are the two electrolyte abnormalities which are very detrimental to cardiac function. Whenever there is metabolic acidosis there is increase in serum potassium to counter the $H^+$ influx into the cells. This hyperkaliaemic effect is more with metabolic acidosis than with respiratory acidosis. Any way acidosis produces hyperkalaemia, which is not good for the heart, it produces myocardial depression and is arrhythmogenic when the level breaches 5.5meq/L. This cardiac depressant effect is only countered by calcium, unfortunately during sick condition calcium levels falls. This is against theory that during acidosis there is hypercalcemia, but in reality, during sick and shock conditions calcium levels always falls. This worsens the toxicity due to hyperkalaemia. So, *my hypothesis is that cardiac depression and arrythmia during shock and arrest all have a common pathway of acidosis, hyperkalaemia and hypocalcaemia induced myocardial depression and arrythmia*. Due to the arrhythmogenic nature of the myocardium it goes into different types of arrythmia, mainly originating from ventricular tissues (VT, VF, pulse less VT). So, reversing the arrythmia and cardiac depression can be done by correcting acidosis, hyperkalaemia and hypocalcaemia. This can be done through the following ways,

- Correct acidosis (metabolic & respiratory acidosis)
    a. Intubate early and use faster IPPV
    b. Correct metabolic acidosis – IV soda bicarbonate
- Correct hyperkalaemia and its effects
    a. Correct metabolic and respiratory acidosis
    b. Counter effects of hyperkalaemia by giving IV calcium
- Correct hypocalcaemia – give IV calcium
- Management of arrythmia
    a. First give IV calcium to counter the arrythmia due to hyperkalaemia
    b. Then specific arrythmia management

c) **Arrythmia induced cardiac arrest (acidosis, hyperkalaemia & hypocalcaemia induced)**

The arrythmia occurring during sepsis, shock seems like a common sequence. There arrythmia is due to multiple causes like electrolyte abnormality (hyperkalaemia, hypocalcaemia, sometimes hyponatremia) metabolic and respiratory acidosis, cardiac myocyte hypoxemia, (sometimes also due to tissue level hypoglycaemia – concept discussed in another chapter). The normal myocytes due to these derangements becomes unstable and easily and spontaneously prone to arrythmia. Arrythmia if not detected or managed properly instantaneously lead to cardiac arrest. In paediatrics 5-10% children take this pathway towards arrest. Of the altered parameters most, important once are the hyperkalaemia and hypocalcaemia. Their correction should also be considered during arrythmia management.

## II. Why was intubation kept at bay (or delayed) in PALS, is it due to difficulty or is it due to lack of necessity?

Frankly speaking neonatal intubation, bag and mask ventilation are easier with little training when compared to paediatric intubation and ventilation. There are more chances of cardiac arrest during paediatric resuscitation. On the other hand, you can maintain oxygenation of a neonate to a fairly longer time with bag and mask and ECM unless complicated by specific causes.

It seems that main crux of the problem in paediatric resuscitation was missed and more importance was given to oxygenation and circulation of coronaries, with no mentioning of blood pH in restoration of cardiac function. Experts may argue that it is very difficult to do a VBG, ABG or a capillary blood gas in this difficult situation. Without knowing blood gas how are we going to manage? In my opinion there is no need to do blood gas as the final common pathway leading to cardiac arrest from shock and sepsis are the same. There will be metabolic acidosis and or respiratory acidosis. First there is metabolic acidosis developing from shock them respiratory compensation sets in and later this compensation fails and both respiratory and metabolic acidosis nose dives the blood pH to lower values. Here if you don't do intubation and faster IPPR you may lose more sicker babies, that may be the reason for the low survival rate for in-hospital paediatric cardiac arrest.

Intubation was not considered early in paediatric resuscitation may be because of the above reason of missing the main point. It is the blood pH correction which should be the priority. Acidosis also causes hyperkalaemia the main depressant of myocardium and inducer of arrythmia. With the same mechanism in mind, you can prevent cardiac arrest by giving soda bicarbonate infusions at an early stage and never allow blood pH to drop below 7.25-7.20 range, at the same time aggressively correcting the primary cause which caused all these problems, that means rapidly upgrading your antibiotics, increasing inotropes or adding new ones. The intubation and administration of IV soda bicarbonate are temporary measures to buy time, if you don't take care of the primary problem the cardiac arrest will come back to haunt you in few hours' time. So, PALS paediatric resuscitation guidelines need a sea change in its approach.

- Preventive aspects towards avoiding cardiac arrest
    - Treat shock aggressively, no harm in over treating shock, but never under treat shock, you will end up in trouble. We should know our limitations, very early detection of shock and complete control of shock is not easy, if there is even a subtle shock individual cells can suffer and each myocyte is a potential timebomb for producing arrythmia.
    - Constant surveillance for detection of shock: BP monitoring, look for tachycardia, bradycardia, tachypnoea, bad coloration for baby, CRT, VBG /ABG/ capillary blood gas, blood lactate, urine output, irritability in a child, cold extremities, uncontrolled seizures, repeat septic work up, worsening pneumonia (X-ray) etc.
    - Do not allow blood pH to fall below 7.25-7.20 range and the safe zone for pH is 7.35 to 7.45. whenever pH dips do the following:
        - Tackle the primary cause, i.e., sepsis by upgrading antibiotics. (new batch of organism can enter from GIT, throat any time into blood stream when you are gravely sick)
        - Increase the dose or add additional inotropes
        - IV soda bicarbonate* to improve blood pH and to by time for other measures to act.

- Elective Intubation if the child is getting exhausted or respiratory compensation is failing i.e., relative respiratory acidosis developing.

- Both intubation and IV soda bicarbonate can bring back the blood pH to near normal and avoid an arrest.

- Take measures to tackle hyperkalaemia and give IV calcium to counter effects of hyperkalaemia

- Hypocalcaemia should be aggressively treated. IV calcium should be a regular drug in sick children.

- Things to do during pre-arrest

  - Intubate and give IPPR at faster rate to wash out $CO_2$, as a compensation for metabolic acidosis.

  - Once you intubate and resuscitate with faster respiratory rate administer IV soda bicarbonate to improve the blood pH, which the body was trying to do but it failed (need not do great things, just follow what the body was trying to do, i.e., use buffers and do respiratory compensation to maintain blood pH).

  - *People arguing against IV soda bicarbonate are discussing internal cellular pH changes, chance for IVH etc are just not justifiable arguments.

  - Do measures to counter hyperkalaemia by giving IV calcium and IV soda bicarbonate (measure to correct metabolic acidosis).

  - IV calcium should be a regular drug during pre-arrest situations.

  - Do all the measures mentioned in preventive aspects of arrest.

> **Role of IV soda bicarbonate in acute resuscitation**
> - To improve blood pH
> - To counter hyperkalaemia
> - To improve buffering capacity of blood (buffering capacity gets exhausted at extremes)

- Things to do during arrest.
    - Immediate bag & mask and ECM
    - Immediate intubation and IPPR (connect to ventilator with higher rate to facilitate $CO_2$ washout.
    - If possible, do VBG /ABG/ capillary blood gas and correct blood pH
    - IV soda bicarbonate once airway is secured or during securing process.
    - IV calcium to revive heart from effects of hyperkalaemia
    - All other measures mentioned in the prevention of arrest.

I wonder how can we avoid doing intubation in a cardiac arrest. All the medical personal and paramedical staff should be trained in intubation of all age groups (neonate, child or adult). Training and perfection should attain during undergraduate period itself. This is only possible by including resuscitation as a practical topic in viva exams. Most of the doctors with PG degree are not confident in neonatal or paediatric intubations not to mention about undergraduates. If doctors don't know intubation, then who are supposed to do intubation?

The regional difference in, paediatric -in-hospital cardiac arrest survival may be due to the difference in the proficiency in intubation.

A doctor witnessing an outside hospital cardiac arrest and not knowing anything to do and patient dying in front of you is the worst experience you can ever encounter. If that unfortunate thing ever happens, then both the system and yourself has to be blamed.

[* *Always give IV soda bicarbonate as diluted solution as slow IV push or as an infusion along with normal saline depending on the acuteness of condition. Even though, soda bicarbonate administration is not officially declared in protocols it is been given in more than 50% of ICU's surveyed*]

**Summary of suggestions in paediatric cardiac arrest**

- Early intubation
- Increase ventilation rate aimed at carbon dioxide washout
- More liberal soda bicarbonate administration after securing airways for bringing up the pH
- Measures to counter hyperkalaemia
- IV calcium to protect the heart
- All MBBS students should be well trained in BLS, ACLS, NALS, PALS. These must be included in the practical exams. Every MBBS graduate should be confident in intubation of any neonate, child or adult.

## CONCLUSION

The above observations are only a hypothesis and more studies are required to establish the facts. The above PALS suggestions are major changes and need studies to disprove or approve. All MBBS doctor should be confident in BLS, ACLS, PALS and NALS guidelines and must be confident in intubations. Intubating a cardiac arrested child is easy compared to a struggling child.

## Chapter 2

# TISSUE CIRCULATION AND PHYSIOLOGY DURING SHOCK AND NORMAL – A DIFFERENT PERSPECTIVE (OXYGEN-GLUCOSE DYAD)

Everybody knows the normal tissue circulation and its regulations and I will be discussing this from a different perspective.

**Normal oxygen transport – what exactly is happening?**

## ALVEOLAR END

Oxygen reaching the alveoli rapidly dissolves into interstitial fluid surrounding the alveoli which then gets into the capillary plasma and from there into RBC plasma and finally get attached to the RBC hemoglobin in a cooperative kinetic manner. This means that there is no direct transport of oxygen from alveoli into the RBC hemoglobin and whatever $FIO_2$ reaching the alveoli has to first get dissolve in the interstitial fluid then into plasma and finally get attached to the hemoglobin, this creates a limitation in the oxygen transport through the blood (may be a protective strategy against oxygen toxicity). Oxygen has very low solubility in plasma and interstitial fluid and the relationship is linearly related. The coefficient for dissolved oxygen transport is 0.0031ml oxygen per mm Hg $O_2$ /dL. The amount of oxygen transported by 100ml of plasma in dissolved form at 100 mm Hg of partial pressure in the alveoli is

= 100 x 0.0031 ml = 0.3 ml of oxygen /dL (room air $FIO_2$ = 21%)

(Amount transported through 15g of hemoglobin is 19.5 ml of $O_2$/dL at a $FIO_2$ of 21%) (Hb vs dissolved $O_2$ = 19.5ml vs 0.3ml dissolved, 98.5% vs 1.5%)

This 0.3ml increases to 2.1 ml of oxygen / dL when $FIO_2$ reaches 100% (700 x 0.0031 = 2.1 ml /dL)

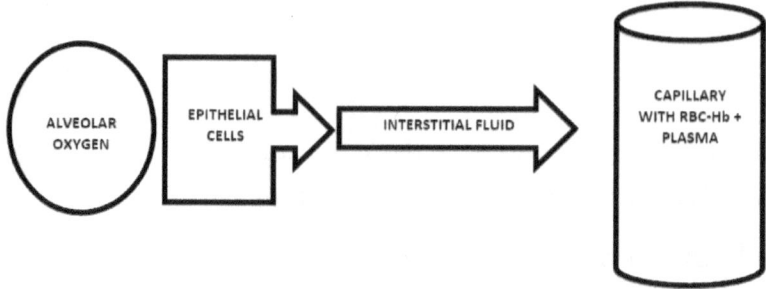

**Figure: 1**  Transport of oxygen from alveoli into RBC

Major portion of oxygen is transported through hemoglobin (98.5%) under room air condition and this decreases to 90% when $FIO_2$ is increased to 100%, the rest 10% is transported through dissolved form. This shows that oxygen carried by hemoglobin (RBC) and plasma is limited by the amount of hemoglobin concentration present. Oxygen transport from alveoli to tissues can be compared to shuttle bus public transport system. Two type of transport can occur in a bus, in seated form and in standing form, seated form corresponds to oxygen carried by hemoglobin and standing corresponds to dissolved oxygen transport. In bus stop there are only standing people corresponding to dissolved oxygen and there the capacity is limited but high turnover is possible provided the bus arrives (Hb) arrives regularly. This oxygen transport from alveoli to hemoglobin in RBC is rapid and it takes only 0.1 second and it happens during one third length of transit through alveolar capillaries (fig: 1 & 2).

## Summary of oxygen transported from alveoli

- Oxygen carried binding to hemoglobin (major)
- Oxygen dissolved in RBC water (negligible)
- Oxygen dissolved in plasma (minimal)

**Table:1**  Amount of Oxygen transported

| Alveolar $FIO_2$ =21% | Alveolar $FIO_2$ =100% | Difference (%) |
|---|---|---|
| $O_2$ carried binding to Hb =19.5ml (98.5%) | $O_2$ carried binding to Hb =19.5ml (90%) | Nil (0%) |
| $O_2$ dissolved in plasma = 0.3 ml (1.5%) | $O_2$ dissolved in plasma = 2.1 ml (10%) | 1.8 ml (8.5%) |
| $O_2$ dissolved in RBC water = negligible | $O_2$ dissolved in RBC water = negligible | Nil |
| Total $O_2$ carried = 19.8 ml (100%) | Total $O_2$ carried = 21.6 ml (100%) | 1.8 ml |
| **Increasing $FIO_2$ from 21% to 100% causes increase of only 1.8ml (8.5%) of additional oxygen transport through 100 ml of blood. Hemoglobin is the real determinant of amount of oxygen transport.** | | |

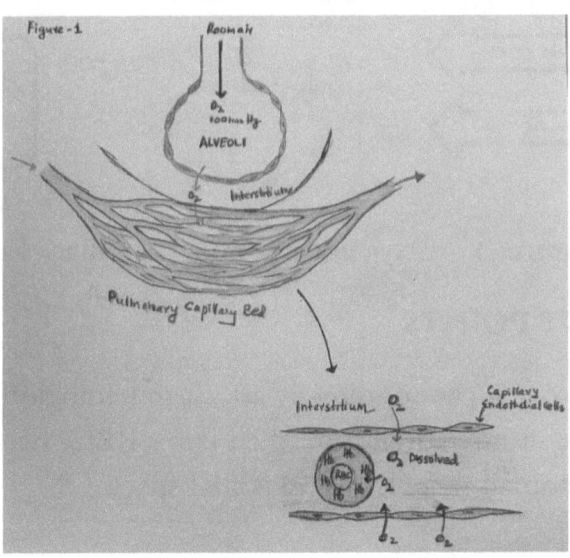

## TISSUE END

As this plasma oxygen and oxygen bound to hemoglobin moves forward it mixes with blood from other areas and reaches heart and distributed to all areas, the dissolved oxygen content and hemoglobin bound oxygen will be same till arterioles and capillary bed are reached. Once capillary bed is reached oxygen diffuses into the interstitial fluid which is continuously and rapidly taken up by the cells. The RBC cannot pass into the interstitial fluid and capillary plasma oxygen is in dynamic equilibrium with interstitial oxygen. RBC bound oxygen cannot be directly transferred into the interstitial fluid or directly into the cells. RBC is continuously supplying oxygen to the capillary plasma and which in turn is supplying into the interstitial fluid from where cells can take oxygen. During this transfer there is no medium which can acts as a reserve for oxygen. Only the RBC can act as a reservoir of oxygen. So as soon as supply is disrupted (during shock) the cells suffers hypoxia.

**RBC – Hb bound oxygen + plasma dissolved oxygen → interstitial dissolved oxygen → cells**

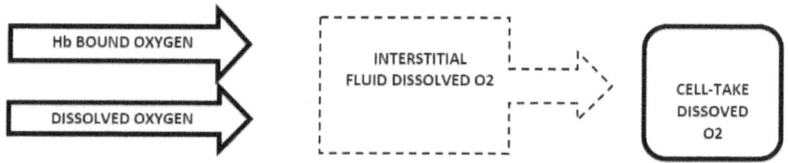

**Figure: 3**   Oxygen transport – Capillary End

## IMPORTANT POINTS

- Alveolar oxygen cannot directly attach to hemoglobin, first it has to dissolve in interstitial fluid then enter RBC. Even though the distance is small there is an interstitial space.

- Alveolar oxygen and dissolved interstitial fluid oxygen concentration is linearly related more over the solubility of oxygen in this fluid is very less. Molecular motion propels oxygen through interstitial fluid into RBC and then attaches to hemoglobin.
- Hemoglobin bound oxygen cannot directly supply oxygen to the tissues
- Hemoglobin bound oxygen just act as a carrier supplying O2 continuously to maintain plasma oxygen tension and interstitial fluid oxygen tension at the tissue end.
- Plasma dissolved oxygen and interstitial dissolved oxygen are in continuous equilibrium
- From interstitial fluid dissolved oxygen cells takes up oxygen continuously.
- **As long as capillary perfusion is good interstitial dissolved oxygen content will be maintained and cells requirement are met.**

## What happens during shock?

Simple definition of shock: it is condition during **which circulation is unable to meet the tissue requirements of oxygen and nutrients**. During shock the preference of body changes, body want to save vital organs at the expense of non-vital organs, so body shunts blood away from non-vital organs (skin, GIT, muscles) to vital organs (brain, heart, kidneys). In the vital organs itself there is preferential allotment to vital centers (brain stem, basal ganglia, grey matter are the compensated area of brain) at the expense of non-vital centers (white matter-non compensated area of brain) (fig:4)

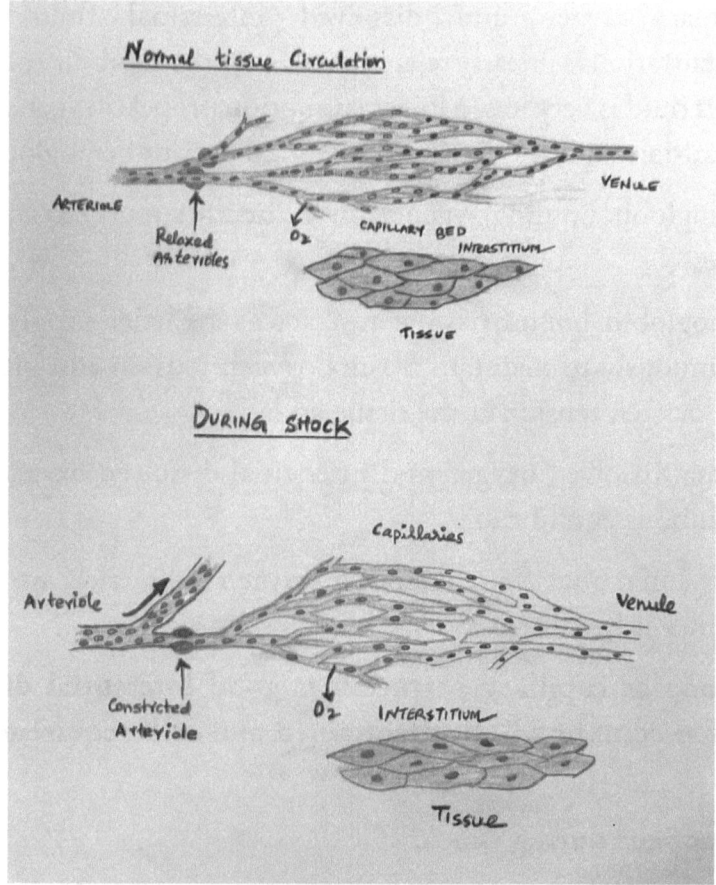

**Figure: 4** Capillary Circulation during Normal and in Shock

At the non-vital organs there is shunting of blood through arteriolar constriction, so less blood flows towards the tissues, this creates an oxygen deficiency and nutrient deficiency in the interstitial fluid. Since there is no oxygen storage capacity for interstitial fluid, in no time whatever oxygen present in the interstitial fluid is used up. It is a dynamic instantaneous deficiency and cells shift to anaerobic metabolism. Most of the non-vital organs (skin, GIT) are resistant towards hypoxia for long periods unless very severe. Muscles and skin are highly resistant to hypoxic damage and they can vary greatly their metabolic requirements. This compensatory mechanism during shock is not foolproof and is not perfect and so it cannot go for long. Vulnerable areas of brain, heart and kidney can suffer. Those areas with highest metabolic demand suffer the most and similarly immature, rapidly growing and multiplying areas of brain. During shock in the brain non vital centers like periventricular white matter suffers most during compensatory or subtle shock. In severe shock any area of brain may get effected.

**During shock, areas of brain can be divided into**

- Compensated areas or vital brain areas (brain stem, basal ganglia, grey matter etc.)
- Non-compensated areas or less vital areas like periventricular white matter

Compensated areas are protected at the expense of less vital areas. During shock bodies priority is immediate survival rather that prevention of long-term neurological deficit. But we treating physicians should be concerned with both, immediate survival and long-term consequences.

My idea of discussion is to bring the importance of subtle shock (subclinical shock) in producing brain damages like that happening in Peri Ventricular Leukomalacia (PVL). There are billions and billions of neurons and supporting cells in the brain, we cannot make sure all cells are well nourished in a compensated or subtle shock situation especially when it is prolonged. Shock in any form need to be treated well, overtreatment will not harm the baby. We have to lower our threshold in detection of subtle shock. If skin color of baby is poor or CRT is prolonged or there is development of mild metabolic acidosis these all means that somewhere body is compromised. These areas invariably are the non-vital areas. Prolonged compromise can produce irreparable damage. There should be no compromise towards shock. Lactate level should never be allowed to raise.

## Normal glucose transport and its compromise during shock.

Glucose is the substrate on which oxygen acts to release energy. Oxygen and glucose should be readily available simultaneously for smooth functioning of the cell so both can be called as oxygen-glucose dyad. Plasma carries glucose and glucose diffuses into interstitial fluid from where cells take it. Problem happens when there is shock. During shock there is blood diversion, less plasma glucose is available for the interstitial fluid and correspondingly less glucose is available to the cells. More during shock due to deficient oxygen supply cells converts to anaerobic metabolism which is highly inefficient and so requirement of glucose sky rockets. Anaerobic metabolism is 18 times less efficient than aerobic metabolism in producing ATP, so in theory cells need 18 times more glucose to do the same work. In non-vital organs (skin, muscles at rest) this may not be a major problem, but this can be a problem in heart, brain and kidneys. In the brain the non-vital areas like brain white matter, periventricular areas suffer "silently" from deficiency of glucose and also oxygen. The word silent is special because there are no surrogate markers for this tissue level hypoglycemia, so mostly it never gets noticed. There are only subtle signs which too are non-specific to tissue hypoglycemia and so usually get attributed to shock. If you check the blood glucose it will be normal but at tissue level there is hypoglycemia due to shock. Subtle signs are irritability, apnea, drowsiness, seizures, USG PVL changes etc. we have to try to find a surrogate marker for tissue hypoglycemia which silently occurs during shock. Till we get a clearer picture and a surrogate marker we have to consider tissue level hypoglycemia along with shock, so try to aim higher blood glucose maintenance level for glucose during shock. This is like giving extra oxygen during shock even if the $SPO_2$ are in the normal range. This may be the reason for the better outcome observed during HIE associated with hyperglycemia.

More detailed discussion is in chapters on shock. This association of silent hypoglycemia accompanying shock is never mentioned anywhere and this seems a new concept having longstanding consequences. If this is proved correct then subtle shock will be taken more seriously and the rush to stop inotropes will not be there. Cutoff value for sugar will be upgraded to higher levels during shock and children will get better neurodevelopmental outcomes. Currently so many neurodevelopmental anomalies like development of PVL, GMH, IVH etc. are only partially explainable due to prematurity. Whatever great you do there is a high chance for the above anomalies to occur. Let this shed light in this area and initiate a larger debate.

**Chapter 3**

# WHICH IS THE MAIN KING PIN IN CELLULAR DAMAGE, SHOCK OR HYPOXIA?

We all know hypoxia and shock can both produce cellular damage. But we are not sure which one of these is deadlier. Over the years we are groomed into believing that hypoxia is the main culprit and always worried whenever $SPO_2$ is in the borderline. Detection of subtle or subclinical shock and its management has always taken a backseat. This is because of the low awareness about the damage it can cause. There is a tendency among residents (reflective of consultants' attitude) to stop inotropes early in a sick child not knowing its consequences. During my practice I run inotropes for longer period until my child is completely out of shock. I am aware that subtle shock is not easy to detect or measure, but can produce havoc if not given due recognition. Neonatology over the years has improved dramatically. In well-established NICU's neurologic outcome is good. In ordinary set up the recognition of shock and management is poor so also their neurologic outcome. In our NICU recognition and management of shock is aggressive. This has led to an excellent neurodevelopment outcome for our babies. Higher grades of PVL, IVH are very rarely seen in our NICUs. I attribute this to the better recognition and treatment of subclinical shock.

How is hypoxia and shock different? Both can produce inefficient delivery of substances to tissues. During pure hypoxia there is adequate blood supply but with insufficient supply of oxygen to tissues. This state is relatively well tolerated by tissues unless $SPO_2$ is extremely low. Congenital heart disease babies can tolerate pure hypoxemia very well without much discomfort. They are comfortable with saturations in the 60's or 70's. Fetus can also tolerate low oxygen levels very well where saturations are in the 20's and 30's. The situation is very different when there is shock, during shock there is low perfusion into the tissues and so, not only oxygen but also glucose and other nutrient delivery to tissues is affected. Shock produces arteriolar constriction and shunting of blood away from non-vital organ to vital organs. In the vital organs also, there is redistribution of blood from non-vital area to vital areas like brain stem. So, in brain areas like periventricular white matter can suffer from ischemic damage.

**Table: 1**   Difference Between Pure Hypoxemia and Shock

| Parameter | Physiology | Cells |
|---|---|---|
| Pure hypoxemia | Oxygen delivery is reduced but supply is still present unless totally cutoff. Technically $PO_2$ of 1 mm Hg is enough for cellular function. (normal tissue $PO_2$ is 23 mm Hg) Glucose delivery preserved | Oxygen deficiency<br><br>Glucose supply normal |
| Shock | Oxygen delivery and glucose delivery to the cells are reduced, during anaerobic metabolism glucose consumption increases. | There is both oxygen and glucose deficiency |

When managing shock don't go by CRT and mean BP alone as these can be deceptive. Mean BP may be last value to fall and you may miss many cases of subtle shock. See for the overall condition of the baby, look for the color of the baby like a dusky colour is a sign of subtle shock. Look for the development of lactic acidosis and see whether sepsis is fully under control. It is better to assume skin perfusion as a reflection of CNS perfusion, if skin perfusion is bad that means CNS perfusion is also bad, incidentally both develops from the same ectodermal tissue.

Shock by definition is inadequate perfusion of tissues there by nutrient supply (oxygen, glucose etc.) are compromised. A cell to function properly nutrient supply should be adequate and so also removal of waste products (carbon dioxide). Main rate limiting nutrients (high turnover nutrients) are the glucose and oxygen. So, whenever there is inadequate perfusion the first to get affected are for the supply of oxygen and glucose. Oxygen deficiency manifests as shift from aerobic metabolism to anerobic metabolism, manifests indirectly as appearance of lactic acid. This cellular shift to anaerobic metabolism is highly inefficient (18 times less efficient compared to aerobic metabolism; 2 ATP produced Vs 36 ATP produced through aerobic metabolism). Due to this inefficiency glucose requirement sky rockets. (approximately 18 times more requirement for the equal amount of work). This glucose requirement cannot be met by the inadequate circulation. So, there will be "local tissue hypoglycemia", which means blood glucose will be normal but at cellular level there will be tissue hypoglycemia, since this is not easy to measure it is easily missed and manifests later as tissue damage. The baby's glucose value may be normal or above normal but there is local tissue hypoglycemia. Body is not able to supply glucose to tissues adequately resulting in tissue level starvation for glucose, starvation in the midst of plenty. How to measure this tissue level hypoglycemia is the next challenge new research into this is needed to find a surrogate marker for tissue level hypoglycemia. (like lactate which is a surrogate marker of anaerobic metabolism). So, when there is shock this local tissue hypoglycemia is marooned by the normoglycemia of the blood. This may be the reason for better neurologic outcome associated with HIE when accompanied by hyperglycemia. This local tissue hypoglycemia produces its worst affects in tissues where metabolism is at the highest, that is in the brain. This "subtle or subclinical shock" produces local tissue hypoxemia and local tissue hypoglycemia which in turn produces neuronal damage. This may be the reason for the high prevalence of PVL, IVH, seizures in neonatal ICUs worldwide. We have to redefine shock and its management to limit the neurologic damage. Shock should be viewed from a different angle, from cellular level, cells are the victims of poor perfusion. Shock should never be measured solely based on the mean BP cut off values. We are not in a position to determine the level of tissue perfusion just by measuring mean BP alone. NIBP can be one of the parameters. Child can maintain BP by secreting counter regulatory hormones, which produces selective vasoconstriction maintaining BP. There should be more eagerness to start an inotrope rather than to stop it. Don't measure shock only through NIBP, mean BP may be the last parameter to fall. Knowing our limitations in measuring shock our cut off for mean BP is always 10 mm Hg higher than the set standard. To compensate for the low tissue delivery of glucose whenever there is shock or "subtle shock" or "poor perfusion" we have to keep the glucose value at a higher level, may be more than 80 mg/dl (need further studies).

When cell is suffering from hypoglycemia how will the cells signal the body to increase glucose supply, or to increase perfusion? What is the cell's panic button? Cell has to convey to the body the difficulties it is encountering. Then only body can take remedial measures. If we can find this link and response then we can detect signs of subtle shock. Is sympathetic stimulation the response of the body towards shock (tachypnoea, tachycardia, hyperglycemia, peripheral vasoconstriction etc.), if so, then we have to give more importance to any of the signs of sympathetic stimulation very seriously.

One of the bodies mechanisms to counter this tissue hypoglycemia is to produce hyperglycemia in the system as a whole. This may be the reason for hyperglycemia seen when there is sepsis and shock. Stress of local tissue hypoglycemia producing hyperglycemia in the child. Local tissue hypoglycemia gets buried in this storm. When this counter mechanism fails to lift blood glucose levels hypoglycemia sets in which is the worst thing that can happen in shock. So, **shock associated with hypoglycemia is a deadly combination for neuronal damage.** When there is tissue hypoxia manifested as raising lactate, or when there is frank shock, you can be 100% sure that there is associated tissue hypoglycemia. That is why whenever baby remains in shock for some time child develops seizures, this is actually local tissue hypoglycemic seizure. Tissue hypoxemia and tissue hypoglycemia go hand in hand during shock. Once cell's energy management goes haywire multiple mechanisms sets in for seizures like accumulation of excitatory amino acids externally. There should be an urgency to over treat shock as we don't know the limit of complete control of shock, there is no harm in over treating shock to save neurons. I always over treat shock and there is a smaller number of seizures in our NICU, and moreover seizures are easily controlled, prescription of long-term seizure medications is extremely less, PVL, IVH, apnea, are all very low in my NICU (15 years' experience). In my experience seizures are better controlled with inotropes than anticonvulsants if you are treating the root cause. That mean it is very difficult to control seizure in sepsis (with subtle shock) with anticonvulsants alone and recurrence of seizure is very common if you don't take care of subtle shock. Recurrence of seizure is almost never seen if shock part and sepsis is well taken care of (anticonvulsant alone = seizure control difficult) ***(anticonvulsant + inotropes = seizure control easy).***

Coming to our chapter topic hypoxemia Vs shock, pure hypoxia as seen in congenital cyanotic heart disease is well tolerated, indicated by non-development of metabolic acidosis, non-stimulation of sympathetic system, non-irritable child (irritability can be a sign of poor perfusion / shock). This happens when there is no associated shock. Fetus are also able to tolerate low oxygen very well. Whenever shock component comes delivery of nutrients (oxygen and glucose) falls precipitously. Oxygen delivery to cells is never direct, that mean, never directly from hemoglobin to cells. In the tissues as blood passes through capillaries oxygen from hemoglobin detaches from it and get dissolved and maintain a particular dissolved oxygen tension in the interstitial fluid and surrounding cells. This dissolved oxygen moves inside cells. Whenever there is shock the continuous supply of dissolved oxygen is cutoff dramatically and cells suffer. Both nutrient supply and oxygen delivery suffers. Whenever there is shock, we never discuss this deficient supply of glucose to cells. This deficient supply of glucose is the damaging part, till not recognized.

In conclusion it is obvious that shock is more dangerous than pure hypoxemia alone. Be very vigilant when you are dealing with sepsis as detection of subclinical shock and its treatment becomes very important. Preservation of all areas of the brain should be your priority. Aim should be "**intact survival**" rather than "**just survival**".

SHOCK IS MORE DAMAGING THAN PURE HYPOXIA

**Table: 2** Progression of shock During Different Stages

| →→ Progression of shock from subtle shock to severe shock →→ | | | | |
|---|---|---|---|---|
| Capillaries | Arterioles | Peripheral artery | Moderately sized artery | Large artery |
| Tissue level | Tissue level | Dorsalis pedis / tibial Radial artery | Femoral / brachial artery | Aorta / Heart |
| Signs and symptoms as shock progresses | | | | |
| Poor skin colour, prolonged CRT | Poor skin colour, Prolonged CRT | Weak peripheral pulses (BP may be maintained) | Weak central pulses (± low BP) | Bradycardia (worst condition, any time cardiac arrest) |

Chapter 4

# CNS MICROCIRCULATION, SUBTLE SHOCK AND BRAIN DAMAGE

Whenever a disease or prematurity happens our first worry is whether there will be long term neurological damages for the baby. I will discuss some practical aspects of brain circulation and metabolism. Brain is a complex organ controlling all other body parts and is composed of billions and billions of neurons and 100 times more supporting cells. Each neuron has 1000's of synaptic connections. The ultimate performance of brain will depend on all these factors. Synaptic destruction, neuronal destruction, supporting cell destruction all will have long term neurologic consequences. Supporting cells are important in myelination and nutrition and overall health of the neurons. If the damage is happening during the early part of development (premature period) the damage is in logarithmic proportion. Destruction of each cell or neuron in the early stage of development results in virtual destruction of thousands of progenitor cells (subsequent generation of cells).

**Loss of cells / Neurons in 1000's**

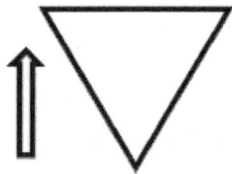

**Single cell / Neuron destruction**

> **Figure:1** Schematic Representation of Single cell Destruction resulting in Multiplier effect

Fetus develops from a single celled ovum and multiplies exponentially. Early damage to the fetus (1$^{st}$ trimester) will be incompatible with life so end in miscarriages. First trimester damage result in severe organ damage as these organs are in the early development phase. Second trimester damage is also severe as organs are still forming. Third trimester damage is less severe unless insult is severe.

**Damage can be grouped into two groups.**

- Like destroying the bud of a sapling
  - Damage can occur for the cells destined to play a major role in future, like the cells destined for migration from germinal matrix. Damage here is unimaginable as whole family of progenitor neurons are destroyed. This is like destroying a bud of a plant.
- Like cutting the formed branches of a tree
  - Damage can occur in the neurons in its final resting place like that in the grey matter, cerebellum etc. This is less damaging compared to the first.

After full term birth neuronal multiplication and cell migration will be continuing till the age of 3 years. By 3 years 95% of the brain growth will be over. Postnatally 70% of neuronal growth and multiplication occurs in the first 7 months of age and 90% of growth will be over by 2 years of age and 95% by 3 year of age. Any insult or deficiency during this period can have varying degrees of long-term consequences. These damages are less severe compared to any damages that occur in the fetal stage. So, practically speaking we have to be very careful in handling a preterm baby, less the maturity more the depth of damage for the same insult.

- When caring preterm babies, we have to be doubly careful

- Not to disturb or stop the normal sequence of brain growth (neuronal proliferation, migration, organization, and myelination). Allow normal undisturbed normal growth.
- Not to destroy rapidly multiplying areas of brain like germinal matrix. This helps in preventing IVH, PVL etc.
- Not to damage already formed areas of brain.

## PLASTICITY OF BRAIN

During brain development there are millions and millions of extra neurons, synapses and supporting cells produced which are subsequently destroyed and is like a remodeling process. This cell death and elimination of neuronal processes and synapses occur during the organizational period of development. It is like that these regressive events are modified when the brain is injured and that neuronal processes and synapses destined for elimination can be retained if needed to preserve function. In addition, new projections can develop in response to injury during the period in which brain has the capacity to carry out organizational events. This process of retaining or preserving neurons and synapses from damaged area is called plasticity of brain and can be seen in pediatric population, for example is pediatric stroke where the normal side takes over the function of the affected side at least partially. Plasticity of brain can be utilized better through early intervention strategies. Earlier you start better the outcome.

## BRAIN CIRCULATION AND VITAL CENTERS.

Brain forms 2% of adult weigh but receives 20% of cardiac output and consumes 20% of oxygen supplied to the body. This shows its huge metabolic demand and 10 seconds of blood supply disruption leads to loss of consciousness and 4 minutes of interruption result in brain damage and 10 minutes stoppage result in complete irreversible brain damage. Brain is supplied through 2 separate set of arteries namely internal carotid and vertebral arteries. All areas of the brain are important but some are more important to sustain life like brain stem and basal ganglia areas. Generally, when body undergoes stress from shock it redistributes blood from non-vital areas (skin, muscles and GIT) to vital areas like brain, heart and kidneys. This is called diving reflex. Here some organs are compromised for the overall survival of the person. Brain gets better blood supply than if there were no diving reflex. But inside the brain, blood is redistributed to more vital areas of the brain (like brain stem, basal ganglia etc.) away from less vital areas like white matter.

But if the shock is sudden like that in cord prolapse or sudden abruption, there would not be sufficient time for the diving reflex to establish and areas of the brain receiving maximum blood supply suffers the most, i.e. brainstem and deep nuclei. Sudden blood supply disruption result in more brain stem damage and gradual and prolonged supply disruption result in more white matter area damage.

Undisturbed glucose and oxygen supply through undisturbed blood supply is the one crucial factor for the normal development of preterm brains. Compromised blood supply is otherwise called shock, and shock is the ultimate destroyer of health of the neonatal brain. Newborns and preterm are highly vulnerable to infection and sepsis and sepsis is the most common cause for shock. Shock can be of different severity and severe shock (uncompensated shock) is easy to identify and difficult to treat and may end in neonatal death. Other type of shock is called compensated shock whereby BP is maintained at the expense of less vital areas. Last variety is subtle shock where compensatory mechanisms has not been initiated but some tissues are compromised.

## TYPE OF SHOCK

Normal classification of shock is compensated shock and uncompensated shock. To get a clearer view on shock we have to zoom these two into

- Subtle shock (subclinical shock)
- Compensated shock (BP maintained at the expense of compensation)
- Uncompensated shock (BP start to fall)
- Terminal shock

**Table:1**  NYLE Classification of Shock

| Grades of shock | Common name | Signs and symptoms | Clinical implications |
|---|---|---|---|
| Grade -0 | Subtle shock | Poor color / dusky color for baby, CRT 2-3, cold extremities, Irritable child, mild metabolic acidosis or mild increase in lactate, apnea seen in pre-terms | Usually misses detection and child can remain in this for prolonged period |
| Grade -1 | Compensatory shock | Tachycardia, tachypnoea, BP increases, decreased urine output, metabolic acidosis & lactate increases, seizures, apnea, desaturations. CRT ≥3 sec, weak peripheral pulses. | Clinical symptoms come up (this is the usual clinical detection stage) |

| Grade -2 | Uncompensated shock | BP start to fall, compensatory mechanisms failed, seizures, desaturations. (central pulsations like femoral & brachial becomes weaker) | Panic stage, rapid deterioration and can rapidly go into cardiac arrest |
|---|---|---|---|
| Grade -3 | Terminal shock | BP falls, bradycardia and cardiac arrest (blood supply to heart compromised) | Hope less period, any time arrest |

**Table: 2** Stages of Shock and Clinicopathological Correlation

| Grades of shock | Micro circulation changes | Damage is to duration & intensity | Neurological implications |
|---|---|---|---|
| Grade – 0 | Arterioles constricts & blood shunted from non-vital to vital organs, tissue level hypoglycemia & hypoxemia, in vital organs blood diverted from non-vital centers to vital centers | Less intense but duration can be longer | Development of PVL, IVH (usually insults are not documented) |
| Grade -1 | Compensatory mechanisms kick in, but microcirculation still suffers | Intensity of shock increases, duration variable | Higher grades of PVL, IVH, brain damage in other areas |
| Grade -2 | Compensatory mechanisms fail | More intense damage | Major damage or +/- death |
| Grade -3 | Total circulatory failure including that for heart | Intense damage | Major damage or +/- death |

## FACTS ABOUT SHOCK

Severity of brain damage is proportional to the severity of shock and duration of shock. So, severe shock of shorter duration produces the same damage as subtle shock of long duration. It is common in NICU to find babies in subtle shock for long duration even for days without recognizing its significance only to produce higher grades of PVL and IVH only to blame on Prematurity. These babies can go into apnea. Babies should not remain in compensatory shock for long (not more than 15-30 minutes) as some areas of the brain are definitely compromised and that leads to damage. Recognizing signs of subtle shock is important for preventing damage.

### How is subtle shock producing brain damage?

Shock by definition is inadequate perfusion of tissues there by nutrient supply (oxygen, glucose etc.) is compromised. A cell to function properly nutrient supply should be appropriate and removal of waste products (carbon dioxide) should also be adequate. Main rate limiting nutrients and high turnover nutrients are the glucose and oxygen. So, whenever there is slow perfusion the first to manifest are the deficiency of oxygen and glucose. Oxygen deficiency manifests as shift from aerobic metabolism to anaerobic metabolism, manifests indirectly by the appearance of lactate and metabolic acidosis. This cellular shift to anaerobic metabolism is highly inefficient (18 times less efficient compared to aerobic metabolism; 2 ATP produced in anaerobic metabolism Vs 36 ATP produced through aerobic metabolism). Due to this inefficient glucose utilization requirement raises proportionately. (approximately 18 times more requirement, for producing an equivalent metabolic performance). This glucose requirement cannot be met by the inadequate circulation. So, there will be "**local tissue hypoglycemia (LTH)**", which means blood glucose will be normal but at cellular level there will be tissue hypoglycemia, since this is not easy to measure this is missed and manifests later as tissue damage. The baby's glucose value may be normal or above normal but there is local tissue hypoglycemia. Body is not able to supply glucose to tissues adequately resulting in tissue level starvation. A situation similar to diabetic mellites, "starvation in the midst of plenty". How to measure this tissue level hypoglycemia is the next challenge. This tissue level hypoglycemia will be maximum where there is maximum decrease in perfusion and in tissues utilizing maximum amount of glucose. But if circulation is not compromised the tissues will get whatever glucose it requires, so damage is seen in areas where circulation is compromised. So, this happens in white matter areas where during shock there is further compromise on circulation. Subtle shock which can remain for long duration can produce havoc here without any dramatic signs and symptoms. The only signs and symptoms may be tonal changes, suppressed reflexes, lethargy, irritability, apnea, or seizures. High resolution USG head at this stage can pick up signals by an expert radiologist. Subtle shock should never be unattended and there should not be any rush to stop inotropes unless doubly sure. (for details see chapter on shock)

## Signs of subtle shock or subclinical shock

- Poor color / dusky color of baby.
- Prolonged CRT, cold extremities, but BP maintained.
- No signs of compensation like tachycardia, tachypnoea or hypertension (No activation of Renin-Angiotensin-Aldosterone axis)
- Irritable child due compromised oxygen and nutrient supply to the brain.
- Mild metabolic acidosis or mildly increased lactate.
- Apnea, lethargy, seizures, depressed neonatal reflexes.

- Feed intolerance (↓ GIT perfusion) sometimes with decreased urine output (↓ renal perfusion)

So, when there is shock this local tissue hypoglycemia is marooned by the normoglycemia of the blood. This may be the reason for better neurologic outcome associated with HIE when accompanied by hyperglycemia. This local tissue hypoglycemia produces its worst affect in tissues where metabolism is at the highest, that is in the brain. This "**unmeasured or subclinical shock**" produces local tissue hypoxemia and local tissue hypoglycemia which in turn produces neuronal damage. This may be the reason for the high prevalence of PVL, IVH, seizures in neonatal ICUs worldwide. **We are underdiagnosing shock and we don't have the specific tool to exactly measure it either**. We as clinicians should speak out our limitations and take a pledge not to undertreat subtle shock. Till the time we invent exact technique to measure subtle shock we should treat or overtreat shock to prevent thousands and thousands of cases of neurologically abnormal babies in NICU's worldwide. If this message is carried across, I am more than satisfied with this book. Our NICU graduate very rarely have grade 3 or grade 4 IVH or PVL. Cystic PVL is almost never seen. But staying in an outside NICU for a week or so produces severe varieties of PVL and IVH prompted me to thing deep into the causes and that led me to uncover these secrets. Various degrees of shock are the secrete separating lower grades of IVH, PVL (1 or 2) from higher grades of IVH and PVL (3 or 4).

Compromised shock is also dangerous but we will be forced to take action because of symptoms and signs. But remaining in compromised shock for long will produce the same damage like that of subtle shock. Always remember damage due to shock is proportional to the severity of shock and duration of shock. A preterm in subtle shock can remain there for prolonged period until it produces dramatic signs or symptoms like apnea, or seizures or till next consultant rounds the next day. This seizure and apnea are due to already initiated neurologic damage. Always treat shock aggressively with volume expanders and with inotropes and take care of the primary reason causing shock which is invariably sepsis. A mild to medium dose of dopamine can do wonders for the baby, color and activity improves dramatically, and also need to upgrade your antibiotics if shock is not parting away.

> **Damage due to shock ∞ to severity**
> **Damage due to shock ∞ to duration**

Of course, there will be people asking where is the evidence, my evidence are my babies treated over 10-15 years of my career. I never started my practice to do any study and at the beginning I never realized the importance of shock and inotropes in brain damage. Over the years I recognized the importance of treating subtle shock. I also noticed less apnea of prematurity (unless extremely premature) for my babies compared to other NICU babies and usage of caffeine is relatively less. This is because I am less afraid of apnea for my babies. Seizures are also less and even if there are seizures continuing anticonvulsants beyond NICU is very rare. I am reasonably confident that my NICU graduates will not have convulsions in future.

Coming to the discussion on shock we have to redefine shock and its management to limit the neurologic damage. Shock should be viewed from a different angle, from cellular level, they are the victims of poor perfusion. Shock should never be measured based solely on a mean BP cut off values. We are not in a position to determine the level of tissue perfusion just by measuring mean BP alone. NIBP can be one of the parameters. There should be more eagerness to start inotropes rather than to stop it. Don't measure shock only through

NIBP, mean BP may be the last parameter to fall. Knowing our limitations in measuring shock my cut off for mean BP is always 10-15 mm Hg higher than the set standard. To compensate for the low tissue delivery of glucose whenever there is shock or "subtle shock" or "poor perfusion" we have to keep the glucose value at a higher level, may be more than 80 mg/dl (need further studies).

## What is the exact mechanism of neuronal damage?

Brain utilizes 20% of cardiac output and 20% of oxygen requirements of the body so also the glucose. Why this much requirement is due to its continuous metabolism to maintain membrane polarity, cellular functions, neurotransmitter production, release and reabsorption. There are 100 times greater number of supporting cells executing various jobs. All require energy. A 10 seconds loss of blood supply produces loss of consciousness. In newborn brain when there is subtle shock in the body the area first effected is the white matter areas where the capillaries carry less blood so also the oxygen and glucose. Brain can revert to alternate metabolites like ketone bodies but they are also cut off due to shock. So, in shock all nutrient supply and oxygen supply is cut that means there is hypoglycemia and hypoxemia. Maximum energy is required for the maintenance of cell membrane polarity through the action of Na-K ATPase. ATP supply disruption causes cell membrane instability, Na+ accumulates inside the cell and K+ outside. Sustained membrane depolarization occurs, **increase intracellular Na causes activation of Na/Ca+ exchange system and movement of Ca+ intracellularly in exchange for Na+** (? mechanism of hypocalcemia in sick conditions). Additional crucial effects of this membrane depolarization are release of excitatory amino acids from synaptic nerve endings and reduced uptake secondary to failure of glutamate transport. The resulting extracellular accumulation of these excitatory neurotransmitters and consequent activation of glutamate receptors result in a variety of deleterious effects, including influx of

Ca+. Calcium also may accumulate intracellularly because of failure of energy-dependent Ca+ transport mechanisms designated to maintain low cytosolic Ca+. The final common pathway to neuronal injury in hypoglycemia is similar to that in oxygen deprivation and relates especially to accumulation of cytosolic Ca+. More over in hypoglycemia, as in HIE, massive depletion of high energy phosphate compound does not appear to be an obligatory event producing cell death.

Considerable data indicate that the mechanism of cell death with HIE is mediated by the extracellular accumulation of excitatory amino acids, which are toxic in high concentrations. It also appears likely that excitatory amino acids play a major role in mediation of neuronal death with hypoglycemia. There are mechanisms for activation of apoptosis during hypoglycemia. Seizure can occur whenever there is shock due to the above-mentioned mechanisms. Sustained membrane depolarization and accumulation of excitatory amino acids are enough to trigger seizure during shock. In clinical practice we can see babies producing seizures and apnea while in subtle shock.

**Take-home message**

- Treat shock aggressively so also sepsis.
- Detect and treat subtle or subclinical shock.
- Staying in compensatory shock is not good for long term neurodevelopment.
- Severity of damage due to shock is directly proportional to the severity of shock and duration of shock.
- Classification of shock bring out subtle shock into limelight.
- Wherever there is shock there is associated tissue level hypoglycemia.
- Utilize plasticity of brain through early intervention measures.

## Chapter 5

# MICROANALYSIS OF PEDIATRIC CARDIAC ARRYTHMIA DURING SEPSIS-SHOCK INDUCED CARDIAC ARREST

(Only discussing cardiac arrest induced by Sepsis -Shock-Sequence)

Cardiac arrythmia is a general occurrence during cardiac arrest especially in adults where main pathology is in the heart. In pediatric population even though it is less (5-15%), it still occurs and in neonatal population it is very less. The order of arrythmia potential is in the following order –adult heart > pediatric > neonatal (seems to follow tolerance of heart towards potassium levels against arrythmia). Neonatal heart is very tolerant to elevated potassium values. Potassium values of 6-6.5 is very well tolerated by neonatal heart but at these values adult heart may shows arrhythmic changes. This resistance towards hyperkalemia may be the reason for the resistance against arrythmia of the neonatal heart. My general view over the years was that cardiac arrythmia was a random event occurring during resuscitation and cardiac arrest and arrythmia can occur at any time. As I learned more and more about the details of events, cardiac arrest and arrythmia seems to follow a common pathway. If they are following a definite pathway then there must be a definite remedy.

My discussion will be around sepsis – shock- sequence related cardiac arrest. Shock and sepsis are a common factor during pediatric cardiac arrest and arrythmia (genetic syndromes related to cardiac arrythmia is not discussed here, for example long QT syndromes). No cardiac arrest occurs during mild shock or mild electrolyte abnormalities. Only when there is severe shock, severe metabolic acidosis, electrolyte abnormalities (hyperkalemia, hyponatremia, hypocalcemia) do cardiac arrythmia occur. So, these factors have some role in its production where one event leading to another. There are definite microlevel causes for arrythmia and our role is to identify these mechanisms. Arrythmia is never a random event. When the myocytes become unstable (due to various reasons like electrolyte abnormalities, acidosis, energy failures) each myocyte is a potential site for abnormal firing.

If you analyze you can see an underline common factor that is acidosis, acidosis leads to hyperkalemia which in turn weakens hearts and it makes heart more vulnerable for arrythmia. More over studies have shown that majority of sick and critical condition is accompanied by hypocalcemia. Hypocalcemia worsens hyperkalemic toxicity; calcium is the one which counters the potassium toxicity. During pre-arrest condition when the bradycardia and inefficient cardiac contractions sets in there is exponential rise in acidosis (metabolic + respiratory acidosis) paralleling that potassium values also shoot up; these changes are impossible to measure at this point ("resuscitation blind spot"). This potassium surge accompanying acidosis suppresses heart further and a vicious cycle of worsening shock sets in. At this tripping point all factors are against heart.

- Worsening blood acidosis (metabolic +respiratory)
- Worsening hyperkalemia
- Worsening hypocalcemia
- Worsening myocardial depression
- Worsening shock
- Myocyte cell membrane instability from ATPase deficiency
- Any time arrythmia

At this moment any type of arrythmia can set in, if that occurs then it can lead quickly towards cardiac arrest. Any counter against these cycles of events is complex. Main culprit to produce arrythmia here is hyperkalemia and actions towards that can prevent or reverse arrythmia. Main weapon towards hyperkalemia is IV calcium and administration of IV calcium should come up in the resuscitation algorithm (better as a prophylaxis). Calcium at this point can counter the effects of hyperkalemia. There is a general misconception among doctors that IV calcium produces bradycardia and cardiac arrest so very afraid to give in a setting of bradycardia. But it may not be true, actually it saves heart from toxicity of hyperkalemia. IV calcium produces better powerful cardiac contractions and helps in overcoming shock. IV calcium stabilizes cardiac myocardium against arrythmia.

**Sepsis -Shock – Sequence leading to Arrythmia and cardiac arrest**

Sepsis & shock → metabolic acidosis → compensatory resp. alkalosis initially → then respiratory acidosis → blood pH drops → hyperkalemia increases → ± hypocalcemia → ± hyponatremia → anytime cardiac arrythmia or cardiac arrest

**Table: 1** Various factors in cardiac arrythmia and its consequences

| Worsening sepsis, shock, aggravating metabolic acidosis, developing respiratory acidosis, increasing hyperkalemia and impending arrythmia or cardiac arrest |||||| 
|---|---|---|---|---|---|
| Primary cause | Blood pH changes | Electrolyte changes | Compensatory mechanisms fail | Arrythmia and cardiac arrest sets in |
| Worsening sepsis and shock | Increasing acidosis (Metabolic acidosis initially, Respiratory acidosis later) | Hyperkalemia Hypocalcemia Hyponatremia | Respiratory and metabolic compensation fails, pH drops very fast, buffering systems are exhausted | Hyperkalemia is the culprit in the development of cardiac arrest and arrythmia. Compounded by the development of hypocalcemia |
| **Remedial measures** |||||
| Control shock and sepsis | Maintain blood pH in normal range: through respiratory & metabolic compensation | Counter hyperkalemia & hypocalcemia through IV calcium | Early intubation and faster IPPR  IV soda bicarbonate  IV calcium | IV calcium gluconate counters hyperkalemia induced changes |

Most of the above measures are a way of buying time rather that definite corrective measures, unless and until the primary causes that initiated all these, that is, sepsis and shock are handled properly arrythmia & cardiac arrest will revisit with more vengeance.

**What are the existing PALS guidelines say?**

| Control shock and sepsis | Not concerned about blood pH and no guideline for correction | No measure to counter hyperkalemia, no advise on IV calcium | No early intubation or faster IPPR, no IV soda bicarbonate or IV calcium | Arrythmias are treated type wise rather than cause wise, here the cause is hyperkalemia compounded by associated hypocalcemia and acidosis |

**End result is uniformly bad**

Pediatric resuscitation seems to be an extension of adult resuscitation proposed by American heart association. In adults cardiac arrest is sudden (MI related) and so there is no shock, sepsis, metabolic acidosis or hyperkalemia. Adapting this directly to pediatrics is a fault. Neonatal resuscitation has escaped from its clutches so the results are relatively better (from experience)

Pediatric resuscitation needs rethinking and new approach, it should be an extension of neonatal resuscitation rather than that of adult

Sepsis and shock are the setting in which metabolic acidosis develops and this sequence slowly goes on to develop myocardial depression, hyperkalemia and cardiac arrest or lead to cardiac arrythmia. Worsening shock and acidosis alter cell membrane Na-K ATPase activity. Shock aggravates cellular nutrient availability (oxygen and glucose) even if saturations are on the higher side. If you are looking only on saturations and BP you may miss subtle shock suffered by tissues (cells suffer hypoxemia and hypoglycemia) but systemic saturations and glucose concentrations are well maintained. Hyperkalemia causes the decrease of resting membrane potential and the membrane becomes partially depolarized. This causes increase in cell membrane excitability. (This sudden increase in membrane excitability occur in acute hyperkalemia and less likely when the hyperkalemia is a chronic process). This increased membrane excitability is the cause for cardiac arrythmia. The most important and only counter to this excitability of cell membrane is calcium. Calcium antagonizes the cardiotoxicity of hyperkalemia by stabilizing the cardiac cell membrane against undesirable depolarization.

Calcium gluconate should be used as the first line agent in patients with ECG changes (sensitivity and specificity of ECG changes during hyperkalemia is poor) or severe hyperkalemia or with arrythmia to protect cardiomyocytes. Other electrolyte abnormality like hyponatremia is less likely to cause arrythmia. But associated hypocalcemia can aggravate potassium toxicity and so IV calcium should be administered during resuscitation with or without arrythmia. If you give IV calcium during resuscitation in patients without arrythmia, it stabilizes the membrane and prevents the occurrence of arrythmia later, cardiac contractions become more powerful and helps in mitigating shock and improves coronary perfusion. In cases already in arrythmia IV calcium counters the arrythmia effects of hyperkalemia and may stop arrythmia.

Once heart is in arrest, metabolic acidosis is only going to increase and also the hyperkalemia. The only way to counter arrhythmogenic effect of hyperkalemia is to give IV calcium gluconate. Chances of arrythmia increases when K$^+$ raises above 5.5meq/L. Once cardiac arrest occurs whatever respiratory compensation was there also ceases (respiratory arrest), respiratory acidosis adds up to metabolic acidosis and blood pH drops precipitously. This sudden drop in pH causes sudden rise of hyperkalemia which is not countered by calcium and so heart is highly prone for depression and arrythmia. These changes are unmeasurable and may not be accurate even if measured or find out from ECG. This is the tipping point towards death. If you can picturize this you can reverse the sequence. The immediate sequences should be, immediate intubation and rapid IPPR, IV calcium gluconate, IV soda bicarbonate and subsequently upgrading of antibiotics to cover all possible organisms (because you won't get a second chance), better shock control by increasing inotropes. Do ABG or VBG and do better control of blood pH. Correct electrolyte abnormalities and closely monitor events.

**Give IV calcium gluconate when there is**

1. Pre arrest like conditions
2. During arrest
3. During arrythmia
4. When there is hyperkalemia.
5. When there is hypocalcemia
6. For any sick child (hypocalcemia invariably accompanies a sick child so always give calcium)

**Changes of ionized calcium status during metabolic acidosis.**

It is known fact that alkalosis is accompanied by hypocalcemia and sometimes even tetany. The reverse happens during metabolic acidosis, that is, there is hypercalcemia during acidosis. But studies have shown that when a child becomes sick invariably there is hypocalcemia. From my experience there are instances of cardiac activity reviving on administration of IV calcium when there was no hope of survival. One baby I remember specifically (near-term 10 days old under treatment for sepsis) went into cardiac arrest suddenly and we continued ECM and bag and mask for almost 10 minutes and immediately after giving IV calcium gluconate child's cardiac activity revived and that baby went home and is now doing well perfectly. There are several such instances were child improved after giving IV calcium gluconate, this observation made me rethink about the mechanisms of cardiac arrest and cardiac arrythmia. It is very difficult to measure the exact values of potassium, calcium or blood pH during these crises. These are dynamic values during arrest and changes rapidly after death and when resuscitation is over. So, measuring exact values and acting accordingly my not be feasible. This blind area is called "resuscitation blind spot" described in detail in another chapter.

So, in short, picturize the blood parameters during sepsis-shock related cardiac arrythmia or arrest. For taking actions exact values are not needed and you can start to do actions one by one and revive the patient and then slowly correct each values based on blood results. One thing to remember is blood parameters are changing rapidly beyond imagination during the terminal minutes of cardiac arrest.

## Chapter 6

# IS SUBTLE SHOCK THE HIDDEN MONSTER IN BRAIN DAMAGE?

**CLINICAL CASE SCENARIO:**

A preterm baby born vaginally at 30 weeks (1.56 kg), was admitted to NICU with mild respiratory distress. Baby was put on CPAP for 48 hour and became off oxygen by day 4 and reached full feeds on day 8 of life. Septic work up was positive and x ray showed few patchy opacites of congenital pneumonia, antibiotics was given for 7 days and no inotropes was started. There were no episodes of apnea, seizures or episodes of hypoglycemia during the stay. This baby was discharged from hospital on 21$^{th}$ day life. USG head done on the day of transfer from NICU showed mild cystic changes of PVL labelled as grade II PVL. This is the usual picture seen in majority of NICUs in the developing countries, all blames put on the prematurity. Is this PVL preventable and my answer is with little bit of more care towards subtle shock this was preventable or reducible in intensity.

Shock has well defined definitions and is always a common factor in critical care ICUs worldwide. Death certificates invariably have shock as one of the sub-diagnosis. We all have over simplified the concept of shock and helped it to hide its ugly face. I doubt whether we are fully seeing the ugly destructive face of shock, the answer is a firm no. Major part of shock is hidden behind the tissue level. We are only seeing the above tissue level face of shock, that is, low BP, prolonged CRT, poor color, development of metabolic acidosis etc. Simple definition of shock is – circulatory system is not able to meet the tissue requirements of oxygen and nutrients. Main tissue requirements are oxygen and glucose, the energy substrate and its igniting fuel. So, everything is about energy requirements for running the cell, that is Na-K ATPase, which consumes the maximum energy. Deficiency of which disrupts cell membrane stability and integrity. Let us picturize shock as an iceberg with parts above water which is known to us and which is below water unknown to us.

## SHOCK THE KNOWN FACTS (TIP OF ICEBERG)

Our discussion of shock will be limited to the shock associated with sepsis. When a baby becomes septic multitude of inflammatory mediators are released by the organism into the system and there are "n" number of counter measures from baby's side. Inflammatory mediators produce leakiness of capillaries and fluid leaks out into the interstitium, producing generalized oedema and hypovolemia inside the vascular compartment. This hypovolemia is countered by secreting chemical which produces vasoconstriction and conserves urine. Kidney start conserving fluid clinically seen as decrease in urine output. BP increases, blood is diverted to vital organs at the expense of non-vital organs. So skin, GIT, muscles get less ration of blood manifested clinically as poor skin color, dusky skin color, prolonged CRT, hypotonia, tiredness, poor GUT circulation may be manifested as poor appetite, nausea, vomiting etc. Vital organs get better blood supply but there is also redistribution of blood supply happening. The blood is preferentially given to vital centers (brain stem, gray matter) at the expense of non-vital centers like white matter. Through these measures baby is trying to hang on to life by preserving function of heart, brain and kidneys. In that process it is compromising function of other tissues which is not important in short term but important in long term. Babies' idea of maintaining BP at whatever expense is to safe life rather than to protect each and every tissues. The counter measures improved perfusion pressure (BP), improved effective blood volume. This state is called compensated shock and is for short term survival as you have an array of tissues who's compromise led to the better perfusion of vital organs. It is obvious that this cannot go for long as these compromised organs start to demand their share or all these compensatory mechanisms crumble on to itself. Converting compensatory shock into uncompensated shock occurs when BP starts to fall and all mechanisms for maintaining perfusion falls and then there is only one way that is road to cardiac arrest.

From this it is obvious that a baby should not be in compensatory shock for long, as you have compromised tissues crying for help. Not seeing their cry is like inviting trouble and later this cry becomes your scream.

## COMPENSATED SHOCK: SIGNS AND SYMPTOMS

- Prolonged CRT, poor skin color, or dusky skin color
- Decreased and concentrated urine.
- GIT upsets like nausea, vomiting, poor appetite, abdominal distension.
- CNS irritability, drowsiness, apnea, sometimes seizures
- Muscle weakness, tiredness.
- Development of metabolic acidosis, increasing lactate, desaturations
- Weak peripheral pulses and near ok central pulses, BP maintained.
- Develops tachycardia, tachypnea, hypertension.

In compensated shock organs can be divided into two sets, **vital organs** (Brain, heart and kidneys) and **non-vital** organs- skin, GIT, muscles etc. non-vital organs compromise for the survival of the vital organs there by overall survival. In the vital organs also, there is redistribution of blood to more vital areas like that in kidneys and brain. In short no baby should be in compensated shock for long, it is a charged time bomb. How long is the question? Have seen doctors not recognizing the subtle signs of compensated shock and happily continuing on compensated shock for long and either ending in collapse or producing long term neurologic damage unknowingly. This is one way of making neurological damage in neonates less in pediatric cases. So, all the following signs should go before we can say there is no compensatory shock.

- No tachycardia
- Normal CRT, BP
- Good color of baby, no cold extremities, child is active not drowsy, no hypotonia.
- No metabolic acidosis, normal lactate
- No irritability for child
- Good urine output.

If you try to avoid all these symptoms that means you are aggressive in treating compensatory shock. What is the role of inotropes? **Inotropes helps to mitigate compensation and allow better perfusion of vital as well as non-vital organs.** So, identify compensated state of shock early and use inotropes more liberally. Always treat the primary cause which caused shock aggressively otherwise shock will return aggressively to haunt you. Better to over treat shock rather than under treat it as you are not able to measure the ongoing damage caused by shock. Simply there are no tools to measure damage caused by subclinical shock.

**ALWAYS REMEMBER**

**Compensated shock = compromised shock = compromised organs = organ damage**

- **Better to over treat shock than to under treat shock**
- **More liberal use of inotropes**
- **Don't rush to stop inotropes**

- **Always be on the lookout for subtle signs of shock**

## SHOCK THE UNKNOWN FACTS (LOWER DECK OF ICEBERG)

Let us go into more microscopic level of shock. Our body is made up of trillions and trillions of cells and our brain the most vital of all contains billions and billions of neurons and supporting cells. Shock effects all cells in the body, some are relatively more resistant to shock and some are highly vulnerable. Neurons are highly vulnerable as they have very high metabolic rate. Constant supply of energy and fuel is a must for smooth functioning. Any interruption in supply is damaging, and shock is the commonly encountered supply disruptor. Even during compensated shock there are plenty of areas of brain which are suffering. Don't be in the impression that during compensated shock all area of brain are well perfused.

**Microscopic view of tissues**

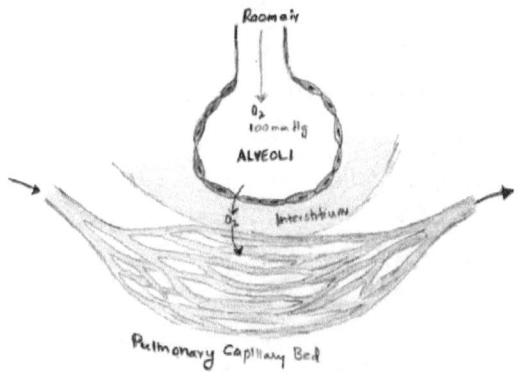

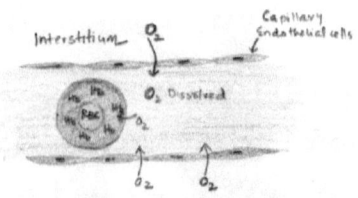

# Barriers and medium in $O_2$ transport

## ARTERIOLAR END

- Arteriole ------- Capillaries ------ endothelial cells ----- interstitial fluid -------- cells

## BARRIERS FROM RBC TO INSIDE CELL

- RBC ---- RBC water ------ Plasma ------- interstitial fluid ------- cell membrane ------ intracellular organelles ------ cell membrane ATPase

## OXYGEN TRANSPORT FROM RBC TO INSIDE CELL

- RBC-Hb bound $O_2$ ---- RBC water $O_2$ ----- plasma $O_2$ ---- interstitial fluid $O_2$ (only form of $O_2$ in interstitium) ------ cells take up dissolved interstitial form of $O_2$ ----- cell membrane ATPase activity

- No direct transfer of oxyhemoglobin to cells (only dissolved interstitial $O_2$ enters the cell)

- No direct uptake of oxygen by hemoglobin from alveoli, always interstitial fluid is an intermediary for all $O_2$ transport. (this may be a protective strategy against oxygen toxicity). The solubility of Oxygen in water is very less so there is no oxygen reserve in interstitial fluid or plasma and so there should be continuous supply of oxygen for cells to remain viable.

- Oxygen uptake and delivery is mediated through interstitial fluid in a dynamic equilibrium, RBC's act like bus carrying oxygen (compressed and crowded, both seated oxygen (Hb bound $O_2$) and non-seated oxygen (dissolved $O_2$ inside RBC).

- At the tissue end dissolved oxygen in the interstitial fluid is the limiting factor for oxygen delivery to cells. When arterioles are constricted there is sudden drop in interstitial oxygen supply, since the solubility of oxygen is very low in plasma (water) the reserve oxygen available is extremely low and cells almost instantaneously experience hypoxemia.

- In analogous to oxygen supply, similar thing is also happening for glucose delivery. Cells also take up the dissolved glucose like dissolved oxygen, so when there is arteriolar constriction glucose supply also stops. So, during shock compensated or uncompensated there is tissue level hypoxemia and tissue level hypoglycemia. During both these instances blood $SPO_2$ and blood glucose levels are normal, decepting the tissue level deficiency. Of these only tissue level hypoxemia produces indirect signs of elevated lactate levels. There are no ways of detecting tissue level hypoglycemia with the present level of technology. We have to assume tissue level hypoglycemia whenever there is shock or whenever there is blood lactate elevation. So, shock means "**tissue hypoxemia-hypoglycemia dyad**", **one is substrate and the other is fuel. It is logic to see when one is unavailable the other is useless**. When glucose is unavailable then available oxygen is useless and glucose becomes useless when oxygen becomes unavailable except when anaerobic metabolism kick starts. When anaerobic metabolism kick starts glucose, requirement shoots up due to the high inefficiency of anaerobic metabolism in producing ATP. Blood lactate levels are a surrogate marker for anaerobic metabolism.

- What will cells do when there is tissue hypoglycemia. They try to utilize ketone bodies as alternate fuel. There is no glucose for lactate production also. Alternate fuel supply of ketone bodies is also in short supply due to the reduced blood supply.

## NORMAL CONDITION WITHOUT SHOCK

Arterioles supply blood to capillaries plentifully and so the arteriolar plasma oxygen content is equal to capillary plasma oxygen content and that is in equilibrium with interstitial fluid oxygen content. This is also true in the case of glucose. Continuous uptake and supply of oxygen and glucose takes place. When the cell requirement increases there is increased supply by arterioles. There are local tissue level regulations for that. This gets disrupted when there is shock.

## DURING SHOCK:

When there is shock their arterioles constricts and blood is diverted, or when there is severe hypovolemia blood reaching periphery will be low (low perfusion pressure). Less RBC flow through the capillaries and also less plasma flow through the capillaries, so availability of $HbO_2$ and dissolved $O_2$ is less, so there is less oxygen in the interstitial fluid, tissues continuously use whatever oxygen and glucose is available and soon end up in short supply. When oxygen supply is exhausted, they shift to anaerobic metabolism and looks for alternate source of energy when glucose is exhausted. So, during compensated shock there is both deficiency of oxygen and deficiency of glucose this can be called **tissue hypoxia and tissue level hypoglycemia**. If you do blood glucose estimation the blood glucose levels will be normal. There is no way to measure tissue level hypoglycemia. When there is tissue level hypoxemia the cells shift into anaerobic metabolism, this has a surrogate marker in the form of lactate which can be easily measured. In short, there is a way to measure tissue level hypoxemia but no way to measure tissue level hypoglycemia. We have to assume tissue level hypoglycemia whenever there is tissue level hypoxemia measured through increasing lactate levels.

During subtle shock or compensated shock blood is diverted from non-vital organs to the vital organs. The blood is diverted from skin, GIT, muscles to heart, brain and kidneys. But the tissues from where blood is diverted don't suffer any damages, because these tissues have very low resting metabolic rates and they are resistant to hypoxic damage. But the brain for which blood is diverted suffer ischemic tissue damage during shock. This is because of its very high metabolic rate. Any damage to neurons or its supporting tissues (oligodendrocytes, astrocytes etc.) will have long lasting consequences. During compensated shock CNS, heart circulations are not perfect and these tissues suffer damage due to poor circulation, this is time dependent, as more the time these tissues experience compensated shock more will be the damage. So, damage due to shock is proportional to the duration of shock and intensity of shock.

**Severity of damage due to shock $\infty$ time duration of shock**

**Severity of damage due to shock $\infty$ intensity of shock**

(less intense shock for long duration is equivalent to intense shock of shorter duration)

So, the following produces same damage:

- severe shock of shorter duration
- subtle shock of longer duration.

This relationship is important because staying in compensated shock is as harmful as severe shock. We tend to take quick action during severe shock as signs and symptoms are more intense and we may lose the patient if no action is taken. We have to be more vigilant and aggressive during compensated shock or subtle shock because the slow damage to cells (neurons) is always masked in the immediate period and manifests only later. This is very important in neonatal intensive care practice. Most damage to the preterm brain may be due to this subtle shock or remaining in compensated shock for prolong periods. During compensated shock vulnerable areas of preterm brain- periventricular areas are deprived of oxygen and glucose and since there is no reserve for these substrate cells undergo tissue hypoxemia and tissue hypoglycemia, which can cause ATP deficiency and can initiate several cellular events like apoptosis. Preterm babies may remain in subtle shock for days {poor skin color, slightly prolonged CRT (2-3 sec), mildly elevated lactate levels, ABG showing mild metabolic acidosis, poor activity, borderline $SPO_2$, occasional apnea etc.}. This creates damage to white matter areas because of compromised circulation, and later presents with varying degrees of PVL, and long-term neurodevelopmental damage. If you take a detail history you will not find any major insulting events. Why this PVL is happening without major events? If any seizure occurs then that is due to more severe cellular damage rather than seizure producing PVL. Insulting events are the same but outcome varies depending on the duration and severity of shock. Subtle damage you may see only milder varieties of PVL and more severe cases produces higher grades of PVL and sometimes produces seizures, apnea tonal abnormalities etc.

For the better understanding of shock, I have categorized shock into 4 grades. Added 2 more grades to the existing classification to get a better view on subtle shock and terminal shock. In the existing classification of compensated and uncompensated shock both ends are blurred and so, subtle shock is merged with the compensatory shock and its features are not clear. Similarly, terminal shock features are not clear, terminal shock has only one direction and that is march towards cardiac arrest and difficult to measure things happens during this stage. These things are exponential rise of acidosis (metabolic & respiratory), rise of hyperkalemia, and hypocalcemia.

## CLINICAL APPLICATION OF SHOCK MANAGEMENT

Shock needs a classification because shock has varied degree of severity, it also helps to highlight subtle or subclinical shock better.

## Table: 1 NYLE Classification of Shock

| Grades of shock | Common name | Signs and Symptoms | Clinical implications |
|---|---|---|---|
| Grade -0 | Subtle shock | Poor color / dusky color for baby, CRT 2-3 or ≥3, cold extremities<br><br>Irritable child, mild metabolic acidosis or mild increase in lactate, apnea for Preterm | Usually missed and child remains in this for prolonged period |
| Grade -1 | Compensatory shock | Tachycardia, tachypnoea, BP increases, decreased urine output, metabolic acidosis increases & lactate increases, seizures, apnea, desaturations (R-A-A axis activation) | Clinical symptoms come up (usual detection stage) |
| Grade -2 | Uncompensated shock | BP start to fall, compensatory mechanisms start to fail, seizures, desaturations | Panic stage |
| Grade -3 | Terminal shock | BP falls, bradycardia and cardiac arrest.<br><br>Exponential rise of acidosis, hyperkalemia, and hypocalcemia. | Hope less period |

**Table: 2** Stages of Shock and Clinicopathological Correlation

| Grades of shock | Micro circulation changes | Damage is ∞ to duration & intensity | Neurological implications |
|---|---|---|---|
| Grade -0 | Arterioles constricts & blood shunted from non-vital to vital organs, tissue level hypoglycemia & hypoxemia, in vital organs blood diverted from non-vital centers to vital centers | Less intense but duration can be long | Development of PVL, IVH (usually insults are not documented) |
| Grade -1 | Compensatory mechanisms kick in, but microcirculation still suffers | Intensity of shock increases, duration variable | Higher grades of PVL and IVH |
| Grade -2 | Compensatory mechanisms fail | More intense damage | Major damage or +/- death |
| Grade -3 | Circulatory failure | Intense damage | Major damage or +/- death |

Most important aim of this classification is to bring a clearer picture about subtle shock which is usually hidden behind the bigger picture. Grade-0 shock is the most important finding of this classification, the facts about subtle shock is already known to everybody but my aim is to bring to the open the damage it creates under the darkness. Grade -0 shock is mostly undetected or not given importance as long as it is not progressing to higher levels of shock. Even though the intensity of tissue hypoxemia and hypoglycemia is low the duration it remains is long to produce major damage in long term. During follow up it may presents as varying degrees of PVL, IVH only to be blamed on prematurity. No major insulting events will be documented. While tapering and stopping inotropes there is a hurry to stop inotropes before full recovery and most doctors maybe stopping inotropes while child may be still be in subtle shock.

For controlling shock, importance should be given for the primary cause which created the shock which is mostly sepsis or hypovolemia otherwise, shock will never get controlled. A shock is fully controlled when you don't have any of its compensatory mechanisms seen. That includes not even slightest of arteriolar constriction. Production of lactic acidosis and metabolic acidosis is a big thing if you dig deep into details. For cellular shift to anaerobic metabolism to occur cells should be under tremendous stress from hypoxemia (and also hypoglycemia). Only a near total hypoxemia can push a cell to death, cells can survive with as low $PO_2$ as 1 mm Hg. In conclusion shock seems to be the silent damager of brain especially in preterm and newborn brains. We have to be extra cautious when dealing with sepsis and shock.

## Chapter 7

# DOES TISSUE LEVEL HYPOGLYCEMIA ALWAYS ACCOMPANY SHOCK? (CONCEPT OF TISSUE LEVEL HYPOGLYCEMIA)

Shock is a common occurrence in ICU's all over the world. Shock is usually associated with deficient supply of oxygen and nutrients, but the nutrient factor is never highlighted or given any importance. Even if discussed only in association with blood level hypoglycemia. Never had the discussion of tissue level hypoglycemia discussed in the setting of blood normoglycemia. If you have understood the full mechanisms occurring during shock from the previous chapters, it is obvious that hypoglycemia invariably accompanies shock. Due to alveolar constriction and diversion of blood there is deficiency of both oxygen and glucose as there are no reserve for these both inside and outside of cell. Oxygen solubility in plasma is very less, so also the available glucose in the plasma or interstitial fluid. Both oxygen and glucose are in dynamic equilibrium with the cellular consumption. Unmeasurable nature of tissue hypoglycemia makes it undetectable or nonexistent. You can assume that if there is development of metabolic acidosis due to poor perfusion then you can be sure that there is also tissue level hypoglycemia. As soon as there is shift to anaerobic metabolism the efficiency of ATP production reduces by 18 times and so glucose requirement shoots up 18 times and supply of that much glucose is not possible in this setting of shock. We can conclude that there is definite tissue level hypoglycemia associated with shock unless proved otherwise.

Roughly $10^9$ molecules of ATP (1 billion molecules) are in solution in a typical cell at any instant and in many cells and this ATP is turned over every 1-2 minutes. So continuous supply is a must in highly active cells and is very much true in case of neurons. That is why damage is instantaneous once there is short supply of blood. Oxygen usage is linked to glucose consumption and as soon as oxygen deficiency causes shift to anaerobic metabolism, the consumption of glucose shoots up due its inefficiency. Meeting the cellular requirements is nearly impossible. Shifting to ketone metabolism is also not possible because in shock its availability is also restricted.

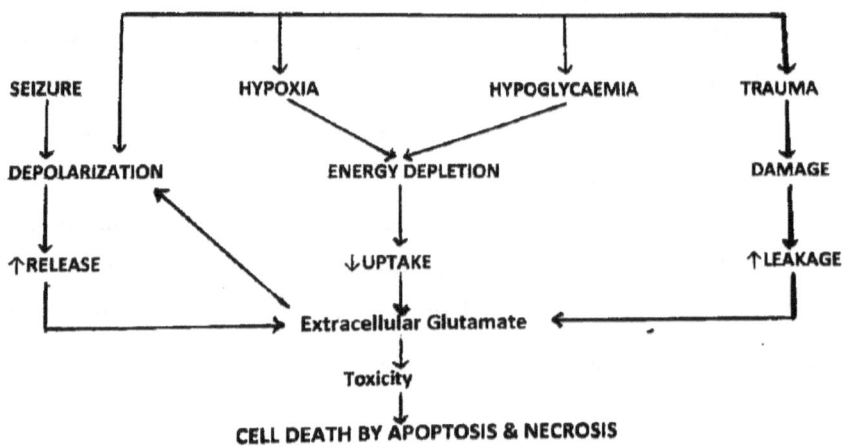

**Figure: 7.1**   Necrotic Cell Death & Apoptosis

| Normal |
|---|
| Oxygen → glucose (4-6mg/kg/minute) →36 ATP (aerobic metabolism) |
| In shock |
| Oxygen deficiency → glucose (limiting factor) → 2 ATP + Lactate (anaerobic metabolism) Metabolism of ketone bodies also limited due to decreased availability due to shock. |

A complete stoppage of blood supply to brain for 10 seconds makes a person unconscious and 3-4 minutes stoppage can result in death. This shows the dynamic nature of the energy and substrate requirements. I wonder why hypoglycemia was never considered during shock. HIE studies had showed us a hint in the form of better neurologic outcome seen in cases with hyperglycemia. We didn't take this leed to its finer analysis. So just higher glucose levels were enough to produce better outcome, this shows the dependency of neurologic outcome on the blood sugar values. If the blood sugar values are higher cells would get a bigger proportion of glucose. It can be assumed that hypoglycemia associated with shock can be a deadly combination.

Hypoxemia and hypoglycemia lead to energy depletion and depolarization of cell membranes. This leads to decreased uptake and increased release of excitatory neurotransmitter glutamate, which in turn causes toxicity to the neurons. Toxicity occurs through apoptosis cell death or necrotic cell death. When the insult is a slow there is more chance for apoptosis cell death to occur and if the insult is acute and severe there is a more chance for necrotic cell death. Excitotoxic amino acid glutamate has a central role in these processes. Both animal and human studies have confirmed this. So, in hypoglycemia and in shock there is both cellular energy deficiency (ATP) and toxicity from excitatory amino acid glutamate. Glutamate toxicity also produces seizure which can aggravate the insult. Seizures further increases energy requirements.

In conclusion treat shock at any cost and consider associated tissue level hypoglycemia with shock. Maintain a higher blood glucose preferably >80 mg/dl when associated with shock. (need further studies to find out the best glucose values during shock).

# Chapter 8

# CAN SEIZURE BE A MANIFESTATION OF SHOCK?

Shock is a common manifestation in neonatal and pediatric practice. There are several causes and mechanisms of shock. Any very sick baby can produce seizure any time. My experience over the years taught me, shock is one of the prominent mechanisms leading to seizures and my strategy of treating shock to control seizures have given great dividend to my babies. In my discussion I am not considering epileptic seizures, febrile seizures or known seizure syndromes. Discussing seizures occurring in ICUs in sick septic children.

## CASE SCENARIO

A 4-day old newborn was brough to NICU with history of respiratory distress, poor perfusion and desaturations and tonic-clonic seizures. Baby was 3.5 kg at birth and was feeding well till yesterday but had mild lethargy. Today morning on rounds was found to have seizures and respiratory distress. Septic work up was positive and x ray showed pneumonic patches. Child had prolonged CRT and NIBP was on the lower side. Treated with IV antibiotics, anticonvulsants, Normal saline push, inotropes and oxygen. Child improved and went home after 10 days, LP done and neuro-sonogram was normal.

## DISCUSSION

This is a usual presentation seen in NICU and all are familiar with this presentation and its management. But this case can be mismanaged in "n" number of ways. Have you ever thought about the mechanism for seizure in such a case?

1. Seizure can occur due to the release of massive amounts inflammatory mediators.
2. Hypoxia to the cells
3. Due to blood hypoglycemia
4. Shock related
   a. Hypoxemia to cells
   b. Tissue level hypoglycemia accompanying shock
   c. Energy failure leading to persistent depolarization of neurons triggering seizures.
   d. Electrolyte abnormalities (hypocalcemia, hyponatremia) also can trigger seizures.
   e. Energy failure leading to the accumulation of excitatory amino acid externally
   f. Apoptosis and necrosis of neurons due to multiple mechanisms

Severe sepsis can cause massive release of inflammatory mediators which can cause seizures. Since LP and USG head are normal, causes related to these are not considered. If you analyze closely all other causes have some relationship with shock. During shock there is diversion of blood from non- vital centers to vital centers. Non-vital centers like periventricular white mater suffers, and in sever shock other centers also suffers. Subtle shock of long duration makes the same damage like severe shock of shorter duration. As explained in other chapters on shock there is energy deficiency to the cells from hypoxemia and tissue level hypoglycemia. Due to the energy deficiency, cell membranes are persistently depolarized, there is decreased uptake of excitatory amino acids, which can trigger seizure.

Apoptosis and necrosis caused by multiple mechanisms also lead to seizures.

In microanalysis of sepsis and shock all shows deficient supply of glucose and oxygen. So, shock is a leading cause of seizure in neonatal and other ICU set up. Early recognition and treatment can prevent seizure, which is usually a late presentation.

## Chapter 9

# REFERRING A SICK NEONATE – A REAL DILEMMA

"In-uteri transport is the best way of transport"

Referring a baby is easier said than done. Lot of practical questions comes in the way, why to refer? when to refer? how to refer? and where to refer? During undergraduate and graduate studies, we all learn in an idealistic way but when it comes to the ground reality it is all different. Initially we try to maintain an idealistic path but over the time we merge with the system. But make sure over the years you improve your system and, on the way, uphold moral and ethical values. We in India will always remain in a resource limited environment, (because of its enormity) that help us to innovate new "Jugaard" ways of doing things, without compromising on patient safety.

Referring a baby from one hospital to the other is a nightmare in our country, wide regional variation in quality of transport is seen but overall, it is a pathetic situation. This is mainly because of the lack of regionalization of care and unavailability of trained manpower and equipments. There are no definite protocols for, whom to refer, when to refer or how to refer. I will be describing my experience from Kerala one of the best states in India when it comes to health care parameters. In tier 1 and 2 cities the condition for neonatal transport is reasonably good still not comparable to western countries. In western countries all the team members (medics and paramedics) are perfectly trained and everybody knows their role. In our country only the doctor will be trained that too imperfectly, nowhere the expert will be accompanying the baby. Over the decades there are major progresses made with regard to transport. The issues related to transport are multitude and varied, can be related to referring hospital, problem related to referring higher center, those related to monetary conditions of patient, availability of training and competency of the transport team etc. General principles of reference are the following.

- If your facilities are inadequate to handle the baby refer immediately.
- Inform and make sure bed is available at the higher center.
- Refer after "stabilizing" the baby, this is the most difficult part.
- Inform parents about the risk during transfer and also risk of not transferring the baby and get informed written consent before transport.
- Transport team should be well equipped and trained.

The idealistic way of transport is not available 90% of the time. Peripheral centers are reluctant to transfer the baby and they refer the baby at the last minute when all options are exhausted. This is because they don't want to lose the customer and don't want to hear the blame of mismanaging the baby. More over there will be pressure from the management regarding why the baby was referred. Some management are satisfied if a reasonable answer is given but some are adamant not to refer any baby. Unless your center is a tertiary care center you cannot treat all the cases under the sky. There can be very sick cases requiring ventilation, HFO, surgical cases, cardiac cases requiring immediate surgery etc. If management is not from the medical fraternity, they may have problem in understanding the situation and nobody should be allowed to play with life. Lots of "management" graduates have "infiltrated" into the system and their sole aim is to meet the monthly targets. This is a bad trend and this tendency should be opposed vigorously. Instead of financial aim they should be concentrating on the patient comfort and patient satisfaction (customer satisfaction).

Always uphold the following in that order:

- Moral ethics and code
- Priority should be 'not to harm the baby" at any cost
- Then comes financial and other aspects

In case of preterm delivery or high-risk delivery if your neonatal team is not in a position to support the baby then it is better to refer the case as in-utero transfer to appropriate centers. This in-utero transfer is highly lacking in our setup. Their aim is to deliver the baby at their center and then refer which is a kind of cheating towards the patient. I have received several 28 weeks preterm babies delivered and then referred, everybody knows the difficulty in managing these babies and the long-term problems they have. Because during transport lots of inconveniences can happen to the parents and lots of additional insults can occur to the baby. Then there is an added financial burden to the parents. Whenever possible do in-utero transfer. In borderline cases of prematurity like 34 weeks, if your team is confident, you can try delivery at your center. Don't deliver 28 weeks at your center and then transfer, it is a nightmare for the parents, for the baby and also for the treating doctor.

If your baby is not doing according to your wishes try to refer the baby at the earliest before any crash occurs. Correct easily correctable things like hypoglycemia and seizures. For shock you can give a normal saline push before referral that can do wonders to the baby. Also put an IV line before transporting a baby, that acts as a life line in case of an emergency. Stabilization of the baby before transport is not always possible because more the time the baby spends in the peripheral center, more will be the deterioration. If the baby is having shock and you are not well trained to handle the shock or facilities restrict you from doing, spending more time is only going to worsen the condition. But can give the basic needs like normal saline push, IV antibiotics and start an inotrope. Most of the ventilators used in advanced level ambulances are of low specifications and are unfit for neonatal transport. Not to mention the technical skills of the technician accompanying.

**Before transport do the following.**

1. Inform the referring center and make sure bed is available.
2. Put an IV line
3. Give IV antibiotics
4. Correct hypoglycemia by giving a D10 push and start on a maintenance IV fluid
5. In shock can give normal saline push,
6. If in shock start inotropes (most peripheral centers won't be starting, 99% of my referred babies didn't had an inotrope during transport)
7. Start oxygen if there is shock, respiratory distress or desaturations
8. If severe respiratory distress or desaturations are present you have to intubate the baby and transfer, this part is not possible by most peripheral centers (from my practical experience). Over the decades this has not changed much, only 10% of cases are referred with ET in-situ. Pediatricians are not confident enough in intubation.
9. If any seizure occurs, start anticonvulsants before transfer, otherwise continuous seizure and any time crash can occur during transport. Neurologic damage from continuous seizures is a reality.

10. If on any continuous IV fluid give fluid through syringe or infusion pump because over or under delivery of fluid can occur if you use a pediatric drip set.

11. Prepare a complete reference letter stating the reasons for transfer, full events starting from antenatal period, and all the treatment given, and the exact condition at the time of transfer.

12. Sometimes tertiary care centers with transport team will come and take the baby, if that is possible then that is the best way of transport.

13. Please sent a reply letter stating the events occurred and diagnosis to the peripheral center. This replay letter is also a rarity in India.

14. Ideal way of transport of neonatologist accompanying with all equipment is not a distant dream, many hospitals have started doing this.

**Examples of worst transport seen. Only 25% of babies are transported "near" ideally.**

- In severe respiratory distress with only nasal oxygen with severe cyanosis and shock with $SPO_2$ of 60 to 70%, they dump and runaway.

- Baby had seizures and referred quickly without any anticonvulsant and reached here with low blood sugar and continuous seizures, you can imagine the outcome.

- Babies reaching in gasping conditions with severe cyanosis and bradycardia on the way to arrest.

- Intubated and reaching with heart rate <60 / min, fully cyanosed with B/L pneumothorax

- Intubated but improperly fixed or ET in esophagus, very much under sized tube. (2.5 ID ET for a 2.5 kg baby).

- Reaching cyanosed and hypothermic
- Bringing dead baby fully covered in cloths, without "monitoring" during transport.
- Cyanosed and in severe shock
- Reaching here with fluid overload and with sever hyperglycemia (GRBS >450mg/dl) from IV fluid infusion without using a syringe pump.

**In India idealistic transport is a distant dream but at least do the following.**

- Wrap the baby properly for temperature control, expose the chest part to see the respiration.
- Do $SPO_2$ monitoring and glucose monitoring during transport.
- Transport with an IV-line, Ryle's tube in-situ, empty the stomach before transport, don't feed the baby during transport of a sick baby, unless you are transporting a very stable baby on full feeds.
- Start a maintenance IV fluid through a syringe pump or infusion pump.
- Check glucose before transport and correct hypoglycemia if any.
- If there is shock, give normal saline bolus and start an inotrope with syringe pump
- Start nasal oxygen if there is desaturations, respiratory distress or shock.
- Intubate if desaturations are severe and respiratory distress is moderate or severe, train nurses not to give too much inspiratory pressure while giving IPPR, co-ordinate with chest rise. Panic comes when there are desaturations.

- Infor the higher center before transport, inform then when you are starting the journey.
- Prevent hypothermia during transport by fully covering the baby or by using a transport incubator.
- If there are seizures ideally control seizures and then transfer, if that is not possible at least start anticonvulsants, if afraid of giving phenobarbitone (given over 30 minutes) because of the apprehension of respiratory suppression, you can give levetiracetam, lorazepam or fos-phenytoin safely.
- Ideally doctor should accompany the transport team, frankly speaking that is not done or possible by most centers. (He or she may be the only pediatrician in that hospital).

In summary, transportation and referral of a baby is a skilled job requiring a coordinated team effort. Whenever possible try for in-utero transport it is the safest, most sterile and cheapest way of transport. We should aim for a western standard of transport in 5 years' time. This requires tremendous improvement in the paramedical undergraduate training, at present their practical training during their course is below standard.

## Chapter 10

# VENOUS BLOOD GAS ON ADMISSION & DILUTED SODIUM BICARBONATE HELPS TO QUICKLY STABILIZE SICK BABIES ON ADMISSION TO NICU

**MY UNBORN PUBLICATION**

A retrospective study was conducted to study the usefulness of venous blood gas on admission and use of diluted Sodium bicarbonate to sick babies admitted to NICU. Study found that blood gas on admission is a good method to quickly assess the seriousness of metabolic derangement. Sodium bicarbonate is useful and safe if used judiciously in late Preterm and term babies.

***Keywords:*** Venous blood gas, Metabolic acidosis, Cardiac arrest

Several babies are admitted in NICU in a very bad condition sometimes even in gasping state. Reviving them quickly and minimising brain damage is a challenge. Chance of cardiac arrest is high during stabilization phase. We have a policy of doing venous blood gas (VBG while putting IV line or UVC insertion) on admission for all babies admitted to NICU [1]. This gives a quick status of metabolic derangement. We also give sodium bicarbonate (1-2ml/kg) diluted slowly to all sick babies admitted. Sick babies include babies with moderate to severe respiratory distress, babies in shock, sick and cyanosed babies, gasping babies, babies in cardiac arrest or babies on the verge of arrest. Additional dose of soda bicarbonate is based on the pH and base deficit. Sodium bicarbonate is given in a dose of 1-2 ml/kg diluted 1:1 with distil water or given diluted along with normal saline bolus over 20-30 minutes [2,3]. We have found this method very useful as we are able to avoid a crash before all medications are started. This helps us to stabilise the babies very quickly. The rationale behind this is that all sick babies have a low pH on admission and low pH (acidosis) results in cellular functional deterioration including that of brain, cardiac muscles [4,5]. Our treatment motto is normalization of blood pH as early as possible and to maintain it, and correction of the primary cause as quickly as possible. With this method we have rarely encountered any cardiac arrests on admission or during resuscitation phase. We have being using this method to quickly stabilize the baby and found to be very useful and so we conducted a 2 year retrospective study of our data.

Two years data (October 2017 to October 2019) was collected from all babies who had received Sodium bicarbonate on admission and from those who had died during this period. The aim of the study is to show the usefulness of VBG on admission (as against ABG, ABG is difficult to collect and more painful) and usefulness of Sodium bicarbonate in stabilizing sick babies on admission [6]. During this period there were 591 NICU admissions [342 (58%) in born & 249 (42%) out born] and there were 16 deaths (2.7%). All blood gas values were VBG from IV line or from UVC.

**Table:1** Data from babies who received soda bicarbonate on admission (n=43) & babies who had died during this period (n=16)

| Parameters | (A) $NaHCO_3$ used & survived (n=35) | (B) $NaHCO_3$ used & died (n=8) | $NaHCO_3$ not used & died (n=8) |
|---|---|---|---|
| Mean weight (Kg) | 2.5 (0.864)* | 1.88(0.786)* *(P < 0.02) | 0.77 (0.147) |
| Mean Gestational age (Wks) | 36.4 (4.6)* | 35 (5.5)* *(P <0.25) | 26 (1.5) |

| Parameters | (A) NaHCO$_3$ used & survived (n=35) | (B) NaHCO$_3$ used & died (n=8) | NaHCO$_3$ not used & died (n=8) |
|---|---|---|---|
| Mean pH on admission | 7.2 (0.14)* | 7.07 (0.22)* *(P < 0.01) | 7.35 (0.07) |
| Mean PaCO$_2$ (mm Hg) | 49.3 (18.7)* | 51.3 (40.2)* *(P <0.45) | 41.7 (11.1) |
| Mean HCO$_3$ (mEq/L) | 18.6 (5.1)* | 12.8 (5.9)* *(P <0.005) | 21.2 (2.0) |
| Mean BE | -8.2 (6.7)* | -11 (13.7)* *(P <0.28) | -4.1 (1.9) |
| Comment on Blood gases | All pH <7.3 | All pH <7.3 | All pH > 7.3 |
| Babies receiving Bag & mask on admission | 8 out of 35 | Nil | Nil |
| Intubation and ventilation on admission (%) | 48.5 % (17 / 35) | 100 % | 100 % |
| Babies getting B & M ventilation or intubation on admission (%) | 65.7 % (23/35) | 100 % | 100 % |
| Mean NaHCO$_3$ use on admission (ml/kg) | 2 | 5.4 | nil |
| Cardiac arrest within 4 hours after admission | Nil | Nil | Nil |

| Parameters | (A) NaHCO$_3$ used & survived (n=35) | (B) NaHCO$_3$ used & died (n=8) | NaHCO$_3$ not used & died (n=8) |
|---|---|---|---|
| Earliest death recorded after admission | No death | 5-1/2 hrs | 14 hrs |
| Neurological outcome (*) | * One near normal<br>* One abnormal<br>* One referred<br>* 91.4% normal (32/35) | All died<br>2 out of 8 died within 24 hours all other died after 8 days | All died<br>only one baby died within 24 hours |

*Values in numbers or mean (SD) (*) Babies with normal tone, angles, breastfeeding well or feeding well with spoon (for preterm babies), with no abnormal movements were considered neurologically normal at discharge from hospital. NaHCO$_3$ = Sodium Bicarbonate*

There were 43 babies (7.3%) who received sodium bicarbonate on admission (table-1). Out of that 35 (81%) survived and 8 (19%) died. Earliest death recorded was at 5-1/2 hours & 19 hours after admission, and all other deaths were after 8 days. There were 8 deaths that didn't received Sodium bicarbonate on admission. These babies were all extreme premature babies with average weight of 770g (147). and average gestational age of 26 (SD 1.5) weeks and their blood gases were all near normal on admission. So they didn't receive any sodium bicarbonate on admission. All survived babies who received Sodium bicarbonate on admission had a pH values below 7.3, with average base deficit of -8.2 (6.7). All babies received an average of 2 ml/kg of sodium bicarbonate on admission and 48.5% babies required intubation and ventilation and 65.7% of babies got some kind of resuscitation on admission. Of all survived babies one was referred, one was neurologically abnormal, one was near normal at discharge and other babies were neurologically normal at discharge (91.4%) (32/37). In the Sodium bicarbonate received but died group average pH on admission was <7.07 (0.22), base deficit was -11 (13.7), they received an average of 5.4ml/kg of sodium bicarbonate. All babies required intubation and ventilation. In the study 76 % (39/51) of babies received some form of resuscitation on admission.

From the study even though most babies were sick on admission there were no cardiac arrest during initial resuscitation phase and most deaths were after 8 days. This shows that blood gas on admission and sodium bicarbonate on admission to selected babies can be of help in stabilizing the sick babies. Sodium bicarbonate administration is safe if given slowly and judiciously and no adverse events were noted. A baby's respiratory distress is due to the sum total of different elements. There can be elements of pneumonia, (Hyaline membrane disease in preterms), elements of PPHN, sepsis, shock, acidotic breathing component contributed by metabolic acidosis. When we are able to decrease this acidotic breathing component of respiratory distress through diluted soda Bicarbonate we are able to bring down the severity of respiratory distress. Shock and other circulatory problems were more easily managed when blood pH is corrected. Without sodium bicarbonate it would have taken hours for the kidneys to correct this acidosis and by that time more and more complications would have taken place. Shock and acidosis are in a vicious cycle were shock worsens acidosis and acidosis worsens shock through poor functioning of all cells including that of cardiac muscles. For any sick baby our aim should be to normalise blood pH as early as possible using Sodium bicarbonate to correct metabolic acidosis or through ventilation to remove respiratory acidosis. This helps the body to normalize functions early. Of course, one has to take care of the primary cause aggressively, otherwise acidosis and respiratory distress recurs and we will be forced to give more Sodium bicarbonate and that may lead to unwanted metabolic derangements and complications. It is a well-known fact that no cardiac arrest occurs when the blood pH is in the normal range.

All cellular enzymatic functions are pH dependent and any deviation of pH from normal will deteriorate cellular functions including that of brain, cardiac and kidney cells [7,8].

Funding: None, competing interest: None stated.

## REFERENCES

1. Kelly, AM, McAlpine, R, Kyle, E. venous pH can safely replace arterial pH in the initial evaluation of patients in the emergency department. Emerg med J. 2001: 18:340-342

2. Usher R, Reduction of mortality from respiratory distress syndrome of prematurity with early administration of intravenous glucose and sodium bicarbonate. Paediatrics 1963; 32 (6): 966-75

3. Afrin M, role of Sodium Bicarbonate to treat Neonatal Metabolic Acidosis: Beneficial or Not. J Bangladesh Coll Phys Surg 2017: 35: 80-85

4. Forsythe SM, Schmidt GA, sodium bicarbonate for the treatment of lactic acidosis. Chest 2000; 117:260-67

5. Shapiro J L, Functional and metabolic response of isolated heart to acidosis: effects of sodium bicarbonate and carbicarb. Am J Physiol 1990; 258:H1835-H1839

6. Kelly, AM. Can VBG analysis replace ABG analysis in emergency care? Emerg Med J. 2016: 33: 152-153.

7. Flemming C, Naoki T, Chikashi T. Distinct pH dependencies of Na+/K+ - selectivity at the two faces of Na K –ATPase. journal of Biological Chemistry, 2018, 293: 2195-2205.

8. Petrus S S, Svetlana N K, Lilia V T, Wolfgang S, Larisa Vasilets. Extracellular pH modulates kinetics of Na K –ATPase. Biochimica et Biophysica Acta 1509 (2000) 496-504

# Chapter 11

# ABDOMINAL PAIN- DOES ULTRASOUND ABDOMEN AND PANIC ALWAYS WARRENED?

Whenever a parent brings her/his child to your clinic with complaints of abdominal pain, there is a panic for parents and surprisingly for doctors also. Is this panic warranted? do we need to do an ultrasound always? These are the questions haunting and compelled me to write this chapter. Doctors are using less and less of clinical skills and logic and going more towards technology. Technology can only assist your decisions and it should not be the sole decision maker. One should thoroughly examine the patient and arrive at a diagnosis. We should never think like parents and we should have the courage in saying that there are no signs for doing an USG abdomen now based on your examination finding and if it is not subsiding or recurring, we will definitely consider. Even if you have a slightest suspicion of surgical abdomen go for USG. Now I have a working diagnosis and see how it responds to treatment.

We should be taking our decisions based on history, clinical examination and basic investigations as and when needed. There is a tendency for unnecessary ultrasound examination whenever a patient presents with abdominal pain. Usual findings seen are the mesenteric adenitis associated with GIT infections. This is like doing CT scan head for all falls. (new trend in the making). Here I want to discuss some of my views and theories about abdominal pain and also want to discuss some usual but unrecognized causes of abdominal pain presenting recurrently for long periods of time.

## Abdominal pain can be divided broadly into

- Surgical causes
  - Infective
  - Non infective
- Non-surgical cause
  - Infective
  - Non-infective
- Psychological causes (very rare in children-but abdominal migraine diagnosis has become more common now a days)

These are the broad classification of abdominal pain, if slightest of doubt is there regarding surgical abdomen, or considering rare pathology, do everything to rule out that. My area of interest is a subgroup of children who present with mild to moderate intermittent colic type abdominal pain which can recur and persist for long duration if not identified and treated properly. The clinical findings in these cases are vague abdominal pain without much localization, sometimes mild cough cold, nausea or vomiting mostly in the morning, sometimes history of recurrent upper respiratory tract infections. There can be a definite onset starting from an episode of upper respiratory infection. On examination one definite finding is congested throat, enlarged tonsils (c/c throat infection), sometimes with nasal block, cold and occasionally presents with abdominal pain with no other symptoms. In short, these silent throat infections can present with abdominal colic and if you treat them properly these episodes subside without much panic. Treatment requires "appropriate antibiotics" as these are unlikely to go away with commonly used antibiotics like amoxicillin or azithromycin. They are chronic cases and are well established. Take a simultaneous throat swab and start with second line antibiotics and if required change to appropriate antibiotics based on culture and sensitivity report. I will be discussing the various mechanisms of abdominal pain for easy understanding.

## MECHANISMS FOR ABDOMINAL PAIN

Gastrointestinal tract starts from mouth and extends down as esophagus, stomach, intestine and ends at anus. Normal function is to accept food, digest it, absorb nutrients and expel waste products. In this complex process there are many supporting organs like salivary glands, lymphoid tissues (tonsils), pancreas, liver etc. to help. GIT accepts food digest it, absorbs it and rest is expelled. It also expels many unwanted materials, unwanted microbes, chemicals, poisons, indigestible materials (plastic, metals) when it enters the GIT. It is fully equipped to deal with all kinds of unwanted things. The whole GIT is fully wired with sensors and can detect any change and deal with it accordingly. The whole GIT is innervated by Vagus nerve and fully wired and coordinated through Meissner's and myenteric plexus. Through these nerve plexus reaches both parasympathetic and sympathetic fibers. For expelling unwanted material or organism it has two processes in hand, one is vomiting and the other is through increasing bowel movements (diarrhea). Whenever an unwanted thing enters GIT (material or organism), immediately it senses it and take action to expel it and the easiest way is to vomit it out. This will be accompanied by nausea. Vomiting is a complex reflex involving coordination from brain, GIT, abdominal musculature and respiratory system. Once the material has passed down into small intestine expelling through vomiting becomes less effective and more difficult. Then GIT alters its strategy and initiate the process of increasing bowel movements.

## COMMON CAUSES OF ABDOMINAL PAIN.

- Intestinal obstruction
- Intestinal infection (gastroenteritis)

- GIT local inflammation (appendicitis)
- Ingestion of indigestible materials
- Cancer and tumor growth
- Liver and biliary tree associated
- Pancreatitis
- Urinary tract infection related
- Females menstrual cycle related
- Worm infestation related
- Gastric and duodenal ulcers (H-Pylori)
- Meckel's diverticulitis
- Simple exaggerated gastrocolic reflex associated with stress or tension
- Psychological – pain abdomen (secondary to some other cause)
- Migraine- recently there is an increased tendency for migraine diagnosis.
- Secondary to chronic constipation
- In breastfeeding babies' due to maternal intake of Ayurvedic medications
- Giving Ayurvedic medications to infants (Vyambu, Bhrami, oil application into the nostril etc.)
- Unhygienic weaning food can cause abdominal pain
- **Undetected or incompletely treated upper respiratory tract infection** (this last one is the most important cause and is always missed as there is no habit of finding subclinical URTI by looking into the mouth with a tongue depressor). This is the whole point of discussion of this chapter.

Unwanted material or organism entry through mouth → GIT senses (receptors) → signals to brain → vomiting initiated → signal to muscles, respiratory center → act of vomiting → material or organism expelled at least partially

## HOW IS THE PAIN PRODUCED?

It is a known fact that >90 % of diseases presenting in the pediatric OPD is related to upper respiratory system. Organism can entre only through mouth or nostril and they will be trapped by the tonsillar lymphoid tissue. Some produce immediate symptoms, some are fully cured, some are incompletely treated, some are forgotten after initial symptoms. Even though URI's are the most common infections the habit of throat examinations with a "tongue depressor" is not so popular among doctors. Without checking throat, the way mentioned you will be missing the current status of infection and complete cure of infection, (details in chapter on upper respiratory infections). The undetected throat infection produces small amounts of mucoid secretions continuously. These secretions are swallowed into the stomach along with microorganisms. Mucoid secretions are indigestible and produces nausea on accumulation. This nausea is maximum in the morning from the accumulated secretions from overnight. Nausea in the child can also manifest as loss of appetite. (when food want to come out how can one take food?) Sometimes nausea ends in vomiting which is followed by some relief for the child. If you closely observe you can see that vomiting will be more pronounced in the morning because of the accumulated secretions in the morning from overnight swallowing. The organisms inside secretions also produce chemical triggers stimulating the nerve endings to produce nausea. Mucoid secretions are not digested inside stomach or intestine. Some amount of secretions pass pylorus and reach small intestine and gets broken down by intestinal bacteria into gas and other intermediates. These produce abdominal bloating and exaggerated peristalsis (exaggerated gastro colic reflex) resulting in colic abdominal pain especially after intake of food or after breastfeeding (typical history is baby cries immediately after starting breastfeeding or child complaints of abdominal pain or have the urge to defecate immediately after taking food). Due to chronic infection in the GIT and due to the action of inflammatory mediator the nerve endings lining the GIT are hypersensitive (like that of nasal mucosa during chronic infections) and produce exaggerated symptoms. Moving digested materials fast towards the anus involves complex reflexes of sphincter dilation and peristalsis. These are the way in which organism or materials get expelled. Normally also continuous peristalsis is occurring without our awareness, that is because nerve endings are not sensitized and we don't feel pain or discomfort. The nerve endings become aware when peristalsis is more intense or more powerful or when the nerve endings are sensitized. This happens when there is obstruction to peristalsis like in intestinal obstruction or when nerve endings are more sensitized due to inflammation from infection. When an indigestible material like a plastic piece is ingested, there can also be fast peristalsis to expel it and, in that process, intermittent abdominal colic is produced. This only last till the material is expelled and this won't take more than 24 to 48 hours.

The constant swallowing of infected secretions produces abdominal discomfort, by producing microfoci of infections throughout GIT, can also produce gas (mucoid secretions). Most USG abdomen at this stage shows only varying degrees of mesenteric lymphadenopathy.

(Always remember GIT starts from mouth and includes oropharynx and all secretions from mouth is dumped into the Gastrointestinal tract. So, any infection in the upper respiratory tract can produce gastrointestinal symptoms).

## How to treat a long duration mild to moderate intermittent colic abdominal pain without obvious localizing signs in a child? (This is a very common presentation in OPD's and never be in a panic to do USG abdomen)

- Take a detailed history.
- Clinical examination includes throat examination with a tongue depressor.
- Take throat swab in all chronic cases and acute non responding cases (it is better to take throat swab during first examination itself)
- Always do urine routine examinations to r/o chronic UTI (do urine culture in appropriate cases)
- If there are throat infections treat it even if it is "asymptomatic". Treat according to symptoms and use appropriate antibiotics.
- Aim for complete cure of infection rather than aiming for symptomatic relief.
- Step up antibiotics appropriately
- Dietary adjustment, if weaning food or other foods are the culprit remove that otherwise symptoms invariably recures (remove the source of infection).
  - In Kerala the culprit foods are: banana-power-mix dried and prepared long ago, Amrutham* powder (health mix, three months shelf life given for a preservative free mix is too long) from anganwadi, grape juice, water melon juice, sometimes mango juice, ice cream, Vyambu and Bhrami given in early infancy). Banana power mix and Amrutham power because of lack of preservatives are prone for contamination easily if kept for more than one or two weeks. It is surprising to see a 3 months shelf life for a baby food without preservatives that too

prepared semi-automatically). Clinically seen lots of infections either diarrhea or respiratory tract infection immediately after starting Amrutham powder (multigrain health mix) even if given for once. Some children adjust it very well. In general, 5 out of 10 children ends up getting some kind of infection. It is best to prepare Amrutham power at home by yourself, lots of you- tube videos are there on how to prepare it.

- A course of deworming can be given (not during acute period)
- Ask for history of pica, habit of pica can produce recurrent throat and abdominal infections. if so, start on iron supplementation and deworming.
- Ultimate aim should be complete cure of throat infection, some may be still difficult because of its chronicity, in that case one or two months of Montelukast after antibiotic course can be given to suppress mucus production and symptoms which can produce symptomatic relief.
- With all these measures, definite cure or a definite decrease in symptoms can be seen.
- After cure avoid foods which can give you fresh throat infections or otherwise you end up in the same vicious cycle.

With the above systematic treatment most abdominal pains disappear, hundred percent there will be decrease in frequency and severity of colic. Do ultrasound only in specific cases to rule out specific causes. Most ultrasounds will only show mesenteric adenitis indicating infection of the GIT. So, there is no need to do USG abdomen in all cases of abdomen pain, use USG judiciously. Most abdomen pain is due to the subclinical and undiscovered throat infections; of course, other reasons are there. Clinically rule out other causes of abdominal pain appropriately.

## SUMMARY:

- Always make a habit of examine throat with a tongue depressor.
- Take a detailed dietary history
- Take throat swab where ever seems appropriate
- Treat URI appropriately and completely, symptomatic relief should not be our aim
- Do USG abdomen judiciously
- Observe everything closely, everything is evolving so also us.

[***Amrutham powder**/ Health mix, is a locally prepared health mix produced under ICDS programme, supplied through Kudumbasree, for children aged between 6 months to 3 years of age. This is preservatives free and has a shelf life 3 months. Shelf life of 3 months seems too long for a preservative free food, from clinical practice approximately 50% of children produce some kind of symptoms of URTI or GIT upset after using it. This is not a study based data but from personal experience. My recommendation is to reduce the shelf life from 3 months to 1 months.]

## Chapter 12

# NYLE TECHNIQUE OF REPLACING BLOCKED PICC LINE WHEN RE-CANNULATION IS EXTREMELY DIFFICULT

Intravenous cannulations are a nightmare in neonatal NICU and less in PICU. This is especially true in extreme premature babies and while treating meningitis cases when repeated cannulations are necessary. We are more depressed when the already working PICC line is blocked in the middle of night. What about replacing it through the same puncture site easily? As the old saying goes "necessity is the mother of all inventions" this is absolutely true in our case. We virtually invented this technique out of necessity. This a very simple and practical technique when your only central line is blocked or when it is time to replace the existing central line or if you want to replace an infected central line and when there is no way of inserting a new central line.

If your PICC line is blocked you will try to flush it with maximum pressure (not recommended) and mostly ends up in failure and you will be forced to put another PICC line. Ideally it is better to put a new one but you can use our method if lines are extremely difficult. It is absolutely sterile and no chance for infection as we are removing all the old catheter and wrappings. I will be discussing replacement of Premicath (28G). Preparations and materials.

**NYLE TECHNIQUE OF PICC LINE REPLACEMENT:**

- All preparations, equipment's and sterile techniques like that for a PICC line insertion.

- Extra materials required: IV canula - 24 G Neocath (yellow), small scissors.
- Remove all the coverings over the PICC line
- Clean thoroughly the catheter and surroundings areas with appropriate sterilizing solutions
- Place sterile towels, exactly like that for inserting new PICC line.
- Procedure:
  - Clean the area of old PICC line insertion site and surrounding area thoroughly with antiseptic solution and allow it to dry.
  - Cut the old Premicath (28G) near its connecting hub.
  - Remove the stylet from the 24 G IV canula.
  - Insert the cut PICC line catheter tip through the plastic IV canula tip using an iris forceps (see figure-1).
  - Pull it completely through its hub
  - Then slowly slide the 24G cannula over the old PICC line through the skin (through old insertion site) into the vein like that of Seldinger technique.
  - Once the canula is inside the vein properly, pull the old PICC line out slowly and take it out and sent the catheter tip for C&S
  - Once it is removed, cut the cannula near its hub using a scissors (figure-1). Using the neocath stylet make the cut cannula opening proper as it would have got compressed upon cutting using a scissor.

- Insert the already prepared new PICC line (28G) through the canula and place it at appropriate length. Once placed slide the canula over the catheter to the other end, clean that with antiseptic solution and remove the blood and clots if any.
- Secure the PICC line properly and start a heparine-saline solution.

- This technique can be used to replace any size PICC line. Always use cannula which is 2 sizes above than of the central catheter. For example,
    - For 28 G PICC line, use 24 G canula
    - For 26 G PICC line, use 22 G canula
    - For 24 G PICC line, use 20 G canula and so on.
- Usefulness of this technique.
    - For replacing blocked PICC line when new canulation is difficult
    - Replacing old PICC line when new canulation is difficult.
    - Replacing infected central line, when new canulation is difficult.
    - For sending infected central line tip for culture and sensitivity.
- This same method can be followed for placing PICC line through a simple IV canula provided the vein is of good caliber. We have place PICC line through a blocked and out IV canula with success.

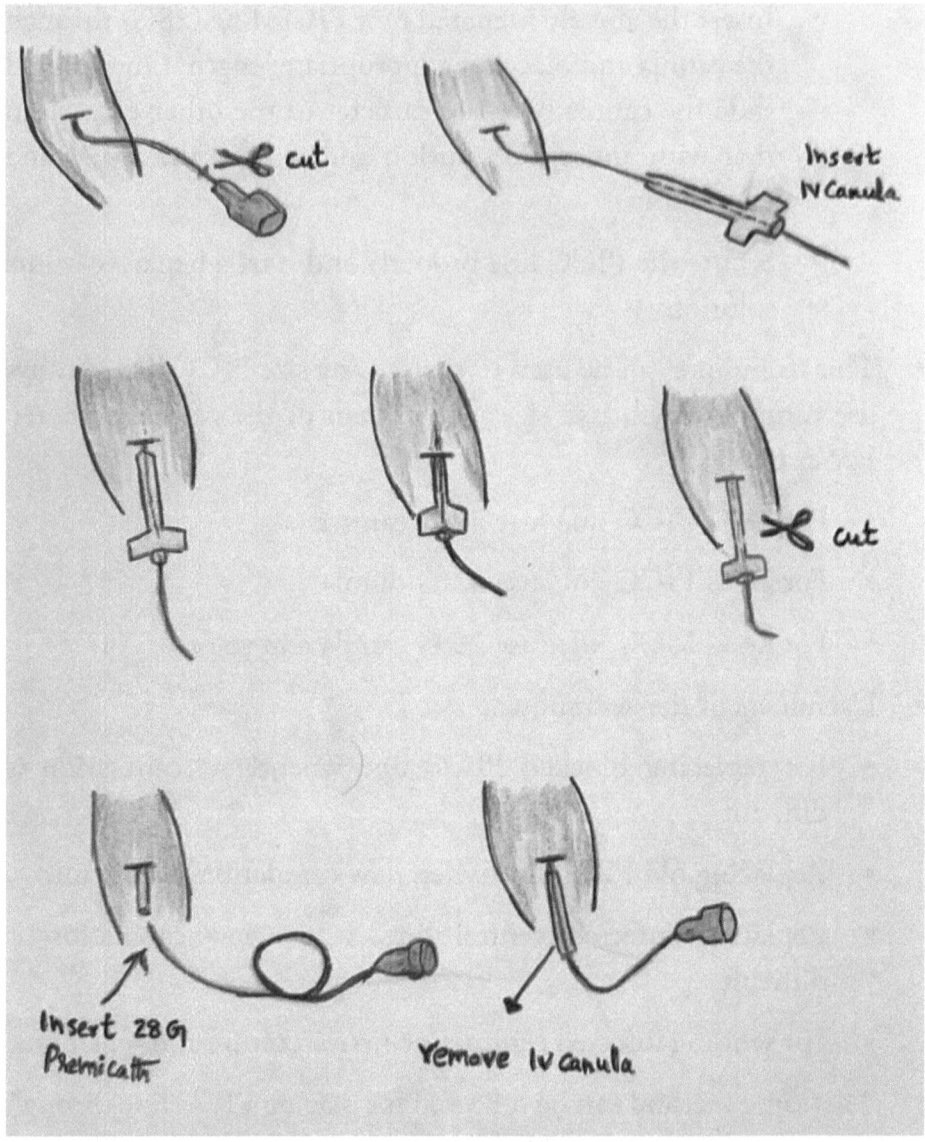

**Figure- 1**   PICC line reinsertion

# Chapter 13

# MANAGING A BABY WITH CRITICAL SERUM BILIRUBIN OF 28MG/DL (HOW TO TACTICALLY AVOID EXCHANGE TRANSFUSION WITHOUT COMPROMISING THE BABY?)

Hyperbilirubinemia is an age-old problem encountered daily in NICU. With the advent of highly efficient LED phototherapy machines hyperbilirubinemia is less of a problem now, more over exchange transfusion has become a rarity. In olden days in large institutions exchange transfusions was a daily event. There is a definite decline in neurologic abnormality cases due to hyperbilirubinemia. It is a rarity to see cases of kernicterus. In spite of all these, cases of hyperbilirubinemia requiring exchange transfusions do come to NICU. The causes of super hyperbilirubinemia coming to our OPD are,

- Early discharge without proper advise for follow up.
- Lack of proper screening of cases into high risk and low risk (SGA, RHI, blood group incompatibility, GDM, lack of screening Serum Bilirubin at discharge)
- Due to associated sepsis.
- Due to undetected rare blood group incompatibility
- Lack of patient compliance, not reporting on follow up date.
- Lack of proper breastfeeding and associated dehydration.

## CASE SCENARIO

A 5-day old FTND baby with a birth weight of 3.2 kg came to the OPD with severe icterus. There is OA incompatibility and serum bilirubin results were 28mg/dl. Admission weight was 2.85kg. How will you manage this baby trying to avoid exchange at the same time decreasing serum bilirubin very fast? Luckily child was neurologically normal, feeding well and active but milk output was low.

Even though this is a case of OAI, there may be added factors which would have precipitated this severe hyperbilirubinemia. What are the factors that can generally trip a child into severe hyperbilirubinemia?

1. Dehydration
2. Infections (invasive and non-invasive)
3. Concealed hemorrhages – cephal hematoma, subgaleal hemorrhage, large contusions etc.
4. Major blood group incompatibility
5. RH incompatibility
6. Minor blood group incompatibility
7. ICT and or DCT positivity
8. Maternal medications
9. TORCH infections

Of these factors the most important and common factors seen in severe hyperbilirubinemia are the dehydration, infection (invasive and noninvasive) and the concealed hemorrhages. If you can take care of these factors quickly you can bring down the need for exchange. Most doctors would have noticed sudden change in complexion for the babies to yellowish color with the onset of infection for NICU babies. Any infection can give a final push towards hyperbilirubinemia.

## MANAGEMENT

Plan of action for this baby is to rapidly decrease the serum bilirubin to less dangerous levels while arranging blood for exchange transfusion.

Anyway, cross matching and arranging of blood takes 2-4 hours. Our aim is to decrease the serum bilirubin to less dangerous level during this time period. Ask the blood bank to cross match the blood and inform us when it is ready and not to issue blood till further orders. Send a second serum bilirubin when the blood is ready, if it has decreased very much continue with current management. Immediately admit the case in NICU, start Double Surface Photo Therapy (DSPT), put an IV Line and do the following,

- Start double surface LED phototherapy
- Start IVF ½ DNS or 10% isolyte -P in the usual rate.
- Give 2 boluses of 10ml/kg normal saline over 60 minutes (total 20ml/kg).
- Send blood for septic work up, electrolytes, urea, creatinine, SBR, SGOT, SGPT, urine RE, GRBS.
- Start IV antibiotics
- Arrange blood for double volume exchange transfusion
- Monitor vitals and neurologic signs at regular intervals
- Send a second Serum bilirubin (SBR) after 4 hours or when the blood is ready for exchange, ask not to issue the blood until further instruction.
- If Serum bilirubin is decreasing reasonably well (decreasing by 3 to 5 mg/dl) continue with current management and if the decrease is only 1-2 mg/dl carry on with exchange transfusion.

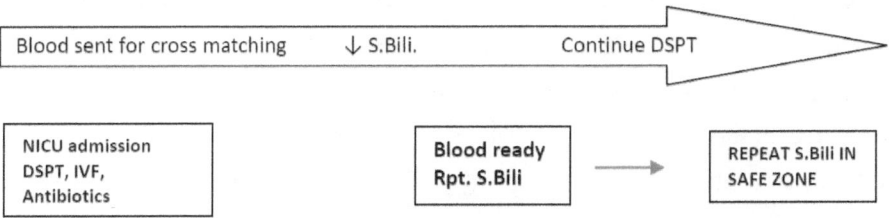

**Figure:1**  Time line of management

In our case serum bilirubin done just prior to exchange transfusion was 22 mg/dl and we continued with double surface exchange transfusion and avoided an exchange. We have managed numerous cases like this and have avoided lots of exchange transfusions and many centers may be using the same technique, those centers who are not using this technique can try and see the difference. Once serum bilirubin is in the safe zone (no exchange needed) you can restart feeding the child (feeding was temporarily stopped to prevent the interruptions in the intense phototherapy and also NBM is better during exchange transfusion). Highest value of serum bilirubin where we avoided exchange transfusion was that of 36mg/dl, where arrival of blood was late due to difficulty in getting crossed matching blood and by that time blood arrived (after 8 hours) we were in the safe zone. This delay was not due the difficulty in getting the correct blood group, but was due to the major incompatibility issue.

## DISCUSSION

In the above case doctors can have several types of management styles, the above method over the years saved me from lots of exchanges and inconveniences for our patients. Usually, most patients get discharged within 48 hours, sometimes even within 24 hours. There can arise several natural questions which needs explanation. Why starting antibiotics before waiting for septic workup? What is the need for antibiotics? When to stop antibiotics? etc.

When dealing with severe hyperbilirubinemia there is only a small window of time for us to play with, that is till the cross matched blood is ready. If you can decrease serum bilirubin to a safe zone during that period then you have succeeded and you can follow your rules, otherwise you have to follow the standard protocol of exchange and continuation of phototherapy. Any baby presenting with severe hyperbilirubinemia have some triggering factors for this exacerbation, triggering factors are,

1. **Dehydration**
2. **Infection – invasive and non-invasive**
3. RHI & Blood group incompatibility- major and minor
4. Hemolytic diseases
5. Other – maternal medications, concealed hemorrhages etc.

Of this most important common factor is dehydration of varying degrees, because during the initial days feeding may not be fully established and milk output is usually low. Giving 2 x 10ml/kg normal saline boluses can bring down serum bilirubin to a certain extend. Other inciting factor is infection, it can be noninvasive or invasive both can trigger hyperbilirubinemia. Septic work up may or may not be positive. Since our window period is less, we have to give it early and not waiting for the result. Our first aim should be to decrease the serum bilirubin to a safe zone. Modern LED phototherapy machines are many times more efficient than old tube lights. More over once you start phototherapy the toxic bilirubin contents comes down drastically, than shown by the total serum bilirubin values. If the baby is septic or if there is RHI then your cut off for doing exchange must be lower, so also when there are suspicious neurological signs. If there are neurological signs then you have to do an exchange even if serum bilirubin comes below exchange level. The point in starting antibiotics early is, if the serum bilirubin raise has anything to do with infection it is unlikely to come down significantly if this infection part is not handled properly. Similarly, in case of dehydration, if it is not addressed properly the bilirubin fall will be very slow. Antibiotic duration depends on the positivity of the septic workup, if septic workup is negative then you can stop antibiotics at discharge.

The above principles can be applied in treating different levels of serum bilirubin.

**Table: 1** Different serum bilirubin levels and action taken

| Serum bilirubin (birth wt:3.2kg, FT) | Actions | Follow up actions |
|---|---|---|
| 34 mg/dl | Triple phototherapy<br>NS Push 20-30ml/kg<br>IV antibiotics<br>IV Fluid<br>Exchange transfusion<br>A complete work up | Continue phototherapy<br>Continue all<br>(Clinical experience has shown better response when there is G+ve coverage*) |
| 28mg/dl | DSPT<br>NS push 20ml/kg<br>IV antibiotics<br>IV Fluid<br>Arrange for exchange (Do exchange, if required) | Continue phototherapy |
| 24mg/dl | DSPT<br>NS push 20ml/kg<br>IV antibiotics (±)<br>IV Fluid | Continue phototherapy |
| 20mg/dl | DSPT<br>NS push 20ml/kg | Continue phototherapy |
| 18mg/dl | DSPT ± NS Push 20ml/kg | SSPT |

\* Seen cases where SBR was reluctant to come down from high levels, came down drastically once MRSA coverage was added.

The total bilirubin level is a sum total of so many contributing factors like, blood group incompatibility (if any), dehydration factor, infection (subclinical or clinical) and if you can deal with each one of them the bilirubin fall can be fast. In the above case if we don't use

IV antibiotics you "may" invariably end up in exchange transfusion. There are things which will not come up in investigations but we have to take it for granted. Sometimes we have to do things (relatively harmless) looking at the big picture.

For junior doctors exchange transfusion may be a rarity. They may be forced to see exchange transfusions from You-tube. Anyway, our olden days of 2 to 3 exchanges on night duty was over and also the occurrence of kernicterus, thanks to the LED phototherapy.

## Chapter 14

# APNEA AS A MANIFESTATION OF EARLY SHOCK

**Can apnea be a manifestation of early shock? Can early inotrope administration prevent apnea?**

In this chapter I will discuss the relationship of apnea and early shock or subtle shock. Definitely shock can manifest as apnea in a preterm baby. By using inotropes early and with appropriate management of subclinical shock apneic episodes can be controlled.

## CASE SCENARIO

A 30 weeks old preterm baby admitted to NICU showed occasional apnea on day 3 of life (already on caffeine citrate) and later the frequency of episodes increased and had to ventilate on day 5 of life. Septic work up turned positive on day 5 even though initial workup was negative. By this time child had prolonged CRT and other clinical signs of shock, inotropes and higher antibiotics was started and child improved and extubated on day 8 of life.

## DISCUSSION:

This is a common scenario seen in NICU and is a clear case of sepsis and shock producing apnea as an early sign. Mostly we take this as apnea of prematurity, but apnea of prematurity should be a diagnosis of exclusion. Apnea of prematurity diagnosis should only be considered after excluding all other causes of apnea. In this case apnea may be the first manifestation of subtle sepsis-shock-sequence and no other signs may not have appeared clinically. Sometimes

Closer look may reveal subtle perfusion deficiencies and septic work up would have prompted early interventions. Starting normal saline push followed by an inotrope and upgrading of antibiotics would have prevented ventilation requirements. Apnea can be a manifestation of early shock; the brain stem vital centers would have undergone subtle perfusion abnormalities and resulting energy failure and accumulation of excitatory amino acids all can manifests as apnea and sometimes as seizures also. Just starting inotropes can prevent further apnea episodes but always take care of the primary cause. If nothing is taken towards sepsis or electrolyte abnormalities the inotrope requirements progressively increases and apnea revisits you. Apnea occurring anytime should prompt a thorough workup including, septic workup, electrolyte, sonogram (+/- LP) etc.

Apnea of prematurity is seen in premature babies below 34weeks. Older babies can also have apnea but due to some definite causes. Babies below 30 weeks can have apnea without other causes and can be rightly called apnea of prematurity, but investigation to rule out other causes should be done. Do other babies with apnea who are >30 weeks has the right to be called apnea of prematurity. My answer is no, because they have some other additional problems which tripped them into apnea. We have to find that cause, mostly it can be shock, sepsis, IVH, PVL, GMH, metabolic acidosis, electrolyte abnormalities, or developing NEC etc. In sepsis and shock apnea can be an early manifestation. In our NICU the use of caffeine citrate for apnea of prematurity is very less for babies >30 weeks. I see apnea as a manifestation of poor brain stem circulation (shock) before other signs appear, of course other causes should be considered. We use more of inotropes for preterm babies rather than caffeine citrate for prevention of apnea. Our incidence of apnea in NICU is very less so also other neurological deficit. This is tectonic shift in thinking and will take year before it can be accepted. I encourage doctors to apply this to patients and see the results. RCT due to so many confronting factors may or may not show up the desired results.

## How is apnea produced?

You have respiratory center in the brain stem controlling respiration. It has afferent impulses (sensory) coming from different areas of brain and from respiratory and cardiovascular system. Based on inputs like blood pH, $PCO_2$, $PO_2$, $HCO_3$ etc. respiratory center controls the respiratory rate and depth. There is a time lag between input and output signals and this is more pronounced in preterm babies. In preterms all centers involved are immature and show waxing and waning effect and any additional insult can precipitate apnea. Due to immaturity any slight insult is enough to derange the functions. Changes like blood pH, perfusion disturbances, hypoglycemia, seizures, electrolyte abnormalities, opening up of PDA and its circulatory changes, sepsis, pneumonia all can lead to apnea. since infection in preterm babies is a common problem, sepsis and shock is a common precipitating factor for apnea, or otherwise speaking you have to rule out infection whenever there is apnea. Due to multitude of factors in preterms subclinical shock is a common accompaniment during infections. Prompt and appropriate action at this stage can save you from more troubles like intubation and ventilation. When apnea occurs rule out other causes and then only label it as apnea of prematurity, otherwise, you are into trouble. In extreme premature babies also before labeling apnea of prematurity rule out other associated causes. In extreme premies perfusion changes can occur even without infections. In preterms because of the immaturity of the respiratory center (myelination not complete, neurotransmitter production and recycling not mature, specific neurotransmitter dominance may not have attained, pathways for input and output signals may not be fully myelinated etc.) it may be highly vulnerable to external influences like pH, electrolyte oxygenation variations, inflammatory mediators etc.

**Respiratory center processing can be affected by different ways**

- Altered perfusion related
  - Sepsis, shock, hypoxemia, tissue level hypoglycemia and energy failure
  - Altered blood pH related respiratory cell depression
  - Accumulation of excitatory amino acid and abnormal firing
- Abnormal afferent impulse from brain (seizure) or periphery (chemical sensory impulse- pH, PCO2, HCO3, PO2, other impulse from GERD, NEC, pneumonia).
- Other systemic insults on respiratory centers
  - Electrolyte abnormalities
  - Hypoglycemia
  - PDA and its hemodynamic effects
  - IVH, GMH, PVL, meningitis

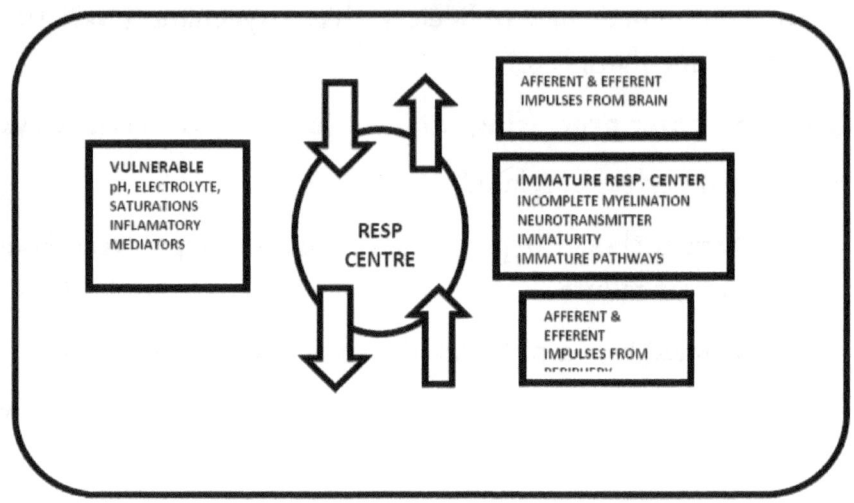

**Figure: 1**  Respiratory center and its vulnerabilities.

Apnea can be a manifestation of "n" number of diseases and my discussion will be restricted to that shock. Most babies in NICU will have sepsis as part of their diagnosis. Apnea of prematurity is a diagnosis of exclusion unless baby is extremely premature like that of 28weeks or less. Other babies if all vital are stable and if there are no signs of sepsis, shock, PDA, NEC, electrolyte abnormalities, IVH, GMH, or PVL should not go into apnea. For these babies any additional insult can push them into apnea. But as the baby becomes more mature, they attain more resistance towards these precipitating factors. After 34 weeks these factors are less likely to precipitate apnea unless the insulting factors are grave. After 30 weeks don't consider apnea of prematurity as the first diagnosis, exclude all factors. While excluding look for subtle shock carefully (poor color of baby, dusky skin, slightly prolonged CRT, mild metabolic acidosis, decreased urine output etc.) because subtle or subclinical shock is a silent cause of apnea. You have to train your eyes towards subtle shock. If you can manage that carefully you can avoid several cases of intubation and ventilations for apnea. Starting a low dose inotrope can work wonders. Subtle shock causes poor circulation of brain centers which trips the child into apnea. So, along with starting caffeine citrate, as a remedial measure look for a cause and start on inotropes (dopamine or dopamine + dobutamine) to improve the circulation. This is very effective way to prevent apnea if you can rule out other definite causes. At the same time tackle the primary cause of sepsis appearing or sepsis worsening by upgrading IV antibiotics. Simultaneously search for other causes of apnea. in our unit we don't routinely start caffeine citrate unless babies are ≤30 weeks. Other babies we use apnea as one of the signs of worsening and treat the primary cause.

Preterm baby's respiratory center is highly sensitive to changes to the blood pH, PCO2, PO2, and electrolytes. So, whenever there is poor perfusion, blood lactate accumulates and pH starts to drop, oxygen deliver decreases all these can alter the respiratory center firing? Cellular function is always dependent on the cell membrane Na-K ATPase integrity. For which circulation and blood pH are crucial. When Na-K ATPase working becomes abnormal, abnormal firing of impulse can occur which manifests as seizures. So, whenever respiratory microcirculation is poor energy failure can occur which can cause apnea and abnormal cellular firing (seizure) can occur early before other manifestations. Controlling shock early and adding inotropes can prevent further deterioration of apnea. Use inotropes for sufficient period of time before sepsis is well under control. These same mechanisms help in better perfusion of other parts of preterm brain and thus can avoid getting PVL, IVH, GMH etc. My unit have very low episodes of serious PVL, IVH, GMH and this may be due to the "over use" of inotropes. Microcirculation abnormality is the real cause of brain damage. There is no direct method to measure microcirculation, now people are using lactate as a marker for that, I use the clinical method of color and appearance of baby, CRT and also lactate levels for development of subtle shock. My practically useful rule is "**if skin circulation is bad, CNS circulation is also bad and if skin color is good then CNS circulation is good**" – after all both develops from ectoderm. If babies' skin is having bad color means babies skin circulation is compromised to make for the CNS circulation, this compensation is not good for long term. If baby is making some compensation means the overall circulation is not good. Help the baby at this stage to tide over the situation. This microcirculation failure can cause apnea in the baby later.

In short apnea can be a manifestation of lots of conditions and one of them is shock especially subtle or subclinical shock. Try out these in your practice to see if any correlation exists.

# Chapter 15

# MANAGING A VERY SICK TERM BABY DELIVERED OUTSIDE AND REACHING YOU IN A VERY BAD STATE

## CASE SCENARIO

A FTND, 2 days old baby was delivered outside and was brought to our hospital in a very critical condition.

## DETAILED HISTORY:

Baby was born to a Primi-gravida mother, FTND, with a birth weight of 3 kg, CIAB, APGAR 8/10 & 9/10 at 1 and 5 minutes respectively gives a h/o maternal fever 2 days back, PROM of 10 hours, Baby had mild grunting immediately after birth and was kept in a not so equipped NICU, started on cefotaxime and gentamycin and gave a 10ml/kg normal saline push and started oxygen at 4 liters/ minute with hood. Initially grunting subsided but tachypnoea and oxygen requirement persisted and on reappearance of grunting at 10 hours of life baby was referred and baby reached us at 28 hours of life with nasal canula oxygen.

## CONDITION OF BABY ON ARRIVAL:

Child was brought to us in a very bad condition. Heart rate 100/ minute, respiratory rate 80/ minute, with grunting, SPO2 82%, CRT > 4seconds, NIBP mean low, cyanosed and dusky, with multiple pricks on the hands and legs with ecchymosis at puncture sites.

**How to manage this baby without much further damage to brain?**

I will discuss this case as a running commentary, problems on arrival, what all problems we can anticipate and what we can do and its logical conclusion behind it. This baby is in severe sepsis, shock (going into decompensated stage of shock), severe metabolic acidosis with respiratory acidosis. Obviously, the next stage is desaturation, bradycardia and crash, how can we prevent the crash and reverse all these abnormalities without much further damage to the brain.

Prepare the bed as soon as the call for reference comes. Took the following vital parameters on admission, HR, RR, SPO2, NIBP, temperature, GRBS, VBG/ABG, admission weight.

**Table: 1**   Prepare the following as soon as we get the call for reference

| Switch on the warmer in manual mode and prepare the bed | Arrange emergency trolley with ET intubation set, AMBU bag, adrenaline etc. |
|---|---|
| Inform, duty doctor, consultant doctor, casualty, reception | Arrange weighing machine, warmer, syringe pumps, suction apparatus, multipara monitor, oxygen flow meter etc. |
| Keep ventilator and CPAP machine ready | |

Assign specific tasks to nurses,

- Nurse for procedure and IV -line insertion and blood collection for investigations
- Nurse for IV fluid preparation and drug administration
- Nurse for taking vital parameters
- Nurse for documentation and other supervision.

**Table: 2** Vitals on admission:

| Vitals | Value | Interpretation & action taken |
|---|---|---|
| Weight | 2.950 kg | Birth Weight 3.2kg |
| Temperature | 36.5*C | Place under warmer |
| $SPO_2$ | 82 % | Start oxygen -hood or nasal |
| CRT | >4sec | Prolonged |
| Heart rate | 182/ mt | Tachycardia from shock |
| Respiratory rate | 80/mt, respiratory distress, Downe's score – 4 to 5 | Start oxygen / SOS CPAP |
| GRBS | 51mg/dl | Hypoglycemia, give D10 push 2m/kg and start IVF |
| NIBP | 58/38/42 | Low mean BP |
| VBG | pH: 7.108, $PCO_2$- 30, $PO_2$- 36, $HCO_3$- 8, BE -16, | Metabolic and respiratory acidosis |

Immediately, IV line was inserted and took VBG, started Normal saline (NS) push 10 ml/kg with added 2ml/kg of soda bicarbonate into the NS push and was given over 15-20 minutes, the same was repeated once more. Second soda bicarbonate dose was decided based on VBG (Venous blood gas) values. Started inotropes dopamine, dobutamine at 0.8ml/mt (16mic /kg/ minute). Started on IV Piperacillin + Tazobactam, amikacin and vancomycin (Must cover most of the ICU organisms including MRSA, MDR gram negative organism). Immediately UVC, UAC was inserted and collect blood for all investigations. D10 push of 2ml/kg was given and started on maintenance IVF 10% dextrose with added calcium, repeated GRBS after 30 minutes which showed a sugar of 74mg/dl. Repeated GRBS at appropriate interval to make sure sugar levels never dip below 60mg/dl. VBG showed severe metabolic acidosis with respiratory acidosis (pH: 7.108, PCO2- 30, PO2- 36, HCO3- 8, BE -16), an additional (2$^{nd}$) 2ml/kg of soda bicarbonate was added to the 2$^{nd}$ normal saline push based on this. After 40 minutes of treatment grunting and retractions decreased, Downe's score came down to 2-3, CRT became <3 seconds, color of baby improved, NIBP improved, oxygen requirement decreased and saturation also improved to >92 %. Chest X-ray showed bilateral pneumonic infiltrates. RT inserted and gastric lavage was given with normal saline, 5 ml mucoid altered secretions was obtained and that was sent for culture and sensitivity.

**Table: 3** Investigation results with interpretations.

| Investigations | Results | Interpretations and action taken |
|---|---|---|
| Hb | 12.5g/dl | Anemia |
| TC | 18,500 | Increased |
| DC | P-80, L-16, E-4 | Neutrophil predominance |
| CRP | 65 mg/L | Increased |
| Platelets | 1.4 L | Decreased |
| GRBS (1$^{st}$) | 51mg/dl | Low |
| SGOT | 60 IU | Mild elevation |
| SGPT | 36 IU | Normal |
| Na+ | 129 meq/L | Hyponatremia – develops as sepsis and metabolic acidosis worsens |
| K+ | 5.3 meq/L | Increasing with sepsis and metabolic acidosis |
| iCa+ | 1.12 meq/L | Lower side |

| Investigations | Results | | Interpretations and action taken |
|---|---|---|---|
| Urea | 27 mg/dl | | Normal |
| Creatinine | 0.9 mg/dl | | Normal |
| Lactate | 80 mg/dl | | Increased |
| VBG pH | 1st 7.108 | 2nd 7.32 | |
| $HCO_3$ | 8 | 15 | |
| $PCO_2$ | 30 | 32 | |
| $PO_2$ | 36 | 38 | |
| BE | -16 | -6 | |
| Cultures sent | | | |
| Throat swab | GPC, GNB – grown MDR Klebsiella | | Send to know the nature of organisms residing. These organisms get into the body during delivery and from NICU. These can invade the body when opportunity arises |
| Umbilical stump | Grown MSSA | | Most probably colonization after birth |
| Blood culture | No growth | | |
| Inguinal swab | No growth | | |
| Gastric lavage | MDR klebsiella grown | | Prenatally or postnatally acquired |

When investigation results came, sodium was 129 meq/L, which was corrected using 3% NaCl. This is by adding half the calculated dose of sodium into maintenance IV fluid over 24 hours and the other half given as bolus over 1 hour. (Sodium correction = 0.6 x weight x (135- serum Na). Sodium value was repeated after 8-12 hours. Continuation of care was given and baby-maintained vitals and repeat investigations was done after 24 hours and the result showed a CRP of 100 mg/L, Na of 136meq/L, K of 47meq/L, VBG was pH:7.34, HCO$_3$: 16 meq/L, PCO$_2$: 38, BE: -5. In view of increasing CRP and dusky color of the baby meropenem was added in a dose of 40m/kg/dose 3 times daily. Child gradually improved over the next 2 days, since there was no RT aspirate for 48 hours, feeding through RT was started at 48 hours of admission. There was no seizure after admission, at 48 hours we removed oxygen, started feeds, tapered inotropes and stopped it after 96 hours, repeated X-ray showed improvement, CRP started decreasing. Started direct breastfeeding by day 6 of life and transported out of NICU on day 8 and discharged from hospital on day 11 of life. child was neurologically normal at discharge. On follow up child was neurologically normal.

## DISCUSSION

In this section, I will be discussing some natural question which can arise from the readers and will give my "logical" answers, this may not be cent present evidence based.

- Is this case referred properly?
- If your NICU cannot handle a case why not refer early?
- Baby would have crashed on its way
- Seizure can occur any time and condition would have worsened.
- Ideally needed intubation before transport but why intubation was not done during transport and why it was not done on arrival?
- What is the idea behind cultures from different sites?
- Possibility of multiple organism entry on its way and during stay in first NICU

- Why does there was no seizure after admission?
- Why used inotropes for such a long period after normalization of NIBP?
- Why used so many antibiotics before getting culture reports?
- Why used soda bicarbonate on admission?
- Why VBG (Venous blood gas) and not ABG done?

**Let us analyze one by one**

Regarding reference of the baby, it was done poorly and done lately. This case would have crashed any time one its way. The referring hospital is also having its own limitations, (discussed in detail all the problems related to referral in an Indian set up in another chapter). You may argue why was not baby referred early. How much early is early? Because of the initial improvement they would have thought that they can manage it by themselves. If they start referring all the distress or tachypneic babies at the initial period itself then they wound be referring most of their NICU admitted babies. They would have missed the secondary deterioration during its initial period, shock was entirely missed, only a well-trained eye can see early signs of shock. Unless nursing staffs are well trained the shock in its early stage can be easily missed. Untrained nurses can only see individual signs and symptoms and they cannot corelate well with the big picture. For example, seeing tachycardia, decreased urine output, occasional desaturations, retractions, grunting etc. has to be taken as a whole and see it as a baby with sepsis developing shock and going into decompensated shock. Your NICU team has to be well trained otherwise you will end up creating your own mess. There is wide gap between early detection and late detection, you may even end up loosing the baby.

Ideally with desaturations and significant retractions you need to intubate and transport. Transport ventilator will be a distant dream for most parts of India, but it will be a reality in the near future. From my experience over the last 15 years, if baby is brought after intubation, managing that baby will be invariably difficult because of very serious infections acquired from unhygienic and multiple failed intubations. Very serious infections with MRSA, MDR or PDR organism would have entered the lungs by that time baby reaches you. So, frankly speaking I am scared of babies coming with endotracheal tubes. Some babies arrive with pneumothorax from over ventilation. These babies will have secondary deterioration after 2 to 3 days after admission. These are deterioration from recently entered organisms. The other side of the coin is, most doctors are afraid to intubate, not able do intubate in a sterile way, sterile techniques usually break down in an intubation panic, equipment and techniques are mostly unsterile, some don't know how to fix the tube around the lips after intubation. Improper fixing is very dangerous because of chance for accidental extubation during transport. Lot of improvements are needed during transport, most are transported in a substandard manner. Resuscitation equipment sterilization is very much substandard in most of the peripheral hospitals. We are not in a position to discard resuscitation equipments after single use, but retrospectively looking that is a far better way economically. We spend lakhs in NICU and save 2000 rupees on bag and mask!

Our baby already got infections inside the uterus (mother had fever 2 days prior to delivery, PROM of 10 hrs.) (PROM- it is premature rupture of membrane before the onset of labor, where infections would have thinned out the membrane and ruptured it). Additional infections would have entered after delivery (from unsterile technique of IV canulation, unsterile NICU environment, multiple punctures, unsterile Labor room, unsterile fluid preparations, unsterile transport etc.) Highly resistant organisms from NICU would have colonized in the throat, stomach, umbilical cord and skin. (NICU colonized organisms are invariably resistant, MDR or PDR organisms or MRSA, MRSE). That is the reason for sending multiple swabs from different sites. By sending multiple swabs from different sites, we will get to know the organisms with which child had contact and these are the organisms likely to enter the baby. These colonized organisms can easily entre the blood stream through mucosal breaks. These colonized organisms (throat, GIT) can enter into the blood stream through intact membranes whenever the host is severely depressed as in the case of shock. In healthy situation also blood stream is constantly seeded by colonized organisms, but these organisms are destroyed by our immune system. But when you are depressed from any stress organisms will gain upper hand and they try to dominate. That is why in most ICU's (MICU, PICU, NICU) the more you stay more higher antibiotics are needed for your survival. All GIT colonized organisms are looking for a dip in your immunity. A severe sepsis, shock, metabolic acidosis etc. are ideal for additional organisms to enter. These late entered organisms take time to multiply and produce symptoms ($3^{rd}$ day deterioration, seen in most ICU's, after admission, initial improvement then around third day there is deterioration unless using higher antibiotics). These kinds of picture may not be seen in the western countries because of the highly sterile techniques used and low incidence of infections in the surroundings. Western countries because of their harsh winter the whole country is sterilized once a year from deep freezing.

When a very sick baby arrives in NICU, we don't have enough time to save the baby without damage. We don't have the time to experiment, that is true in case of antibiotic usage. There is no time to see whether our $1^{st}$ or $2^{nd}$ line antibiotics will work or not. In this juncture you have to hit the nail over its head. At the initial presentation itself we have to cover all types of organism namely G+ve, G-ve organisms resistant organisms. Main one's are methicillin resistant gram-positive organisms (MRSA or MRSE) and MDR or PDR gram negative organisms and ESBL producers. Main NICU culprits are Klebsiella, E-Coli, Pseudomonas, Acinetobacter, MRSA and MRSE. This was the logic behind starting multiple antibiotics, to cover most of the potential organisms.

**General treatment TRIAD of PNM**

(Hit **Primary insult**, **Normalize** altered parameters and **Maintain** parameters)

- Hit the **Primary insult**.
- **Normalize** all body parameters as early as possible (can be cause secondary damages) (Perfusion, pH, Na, K, Ca, GRBS, NIBP, $SPO_2$ etc.)
- **Maintain** the normalized parameters in its normal range.

The above plan of action can be taken for treating any diseases. First identify the **Primary cause** which started all these, treat that without fail. The primary cause is mostly infections sometimes it can be asphyxia with infections, sometimes severe blood loss causing shock etc. Primary cause can be multiple also, try to identify that as early as possible, for example, asphyxia and infections. Then try to bring back all the altered parameters to near normal as early as possible, called Normalization. Utmost priority should be given to blood pH variations because this affects all the cellular functions of all cells especially that of neurons and cardiac myocytes. A severe acidosis depresses all cells, all cellular functions are depressed, it produces hyperkalemia which depresses cardiac myocytes and promotes cardiac arrythmia. Depressed cardiac myocytes cause more shock and a deadly vicious cycle sets in.

The parameters which need immediate attention are blood pH related, electrolytes (Na, K, Ca), blood sugar, shock, anemia, saturations etc. Once the altered parameters are normalized body regains its strength to fight infections. The next step is to **Maintain** these altered parameters in the normal range and prevent slippage of any parameters into the abnormal range (so need surveillance). No need to do big things, if good environment is created most of the time body itself can bring back all altered parameters to normal. Any parameters remaining in abnormal range for long can produce damage, for example, hypoglycemia, hyponatremia, if prolonged they can cause seizures and brain damage. The problem comes when there is laziness in bring back the altered parameters or when the primary cause is not tackled properly. If our baby remained in shock or metabolic acidosis for long then this baby would been on ventilator, would have produced seizures, these all can produce severe brain damage. If infection is not tackled properly then the shock will remain and brain damage and seizure would ensure. Tackle primary cause on a war footing scale, a war footing scale, whatever may be the cost. One thing to remember is correction of parameters may be very difficult if you fail to control the primary insult, like for example if there is hyponatremia or shock controlling these will be extremely difficult if you fail to control the infection which is the primary cause (figure-1).

So, in our case do the following (PNM):

1. Treat **Primary cause,** that is, infection aggressively.

2. Bring back all the abnormal values to the normal (Normalization).

    a. Glucose, shock, sodium, blood gas parameters, saturations, temperature etc.

3. **Maintain** all normalized parameters and prevent slippage of any parameters

a. Prevent hypocalcemia, hypernatremia, hyperkalemia, acidosis, shock etc.
4. Be in constant vigil against any additional insults or slippage of any parameters.

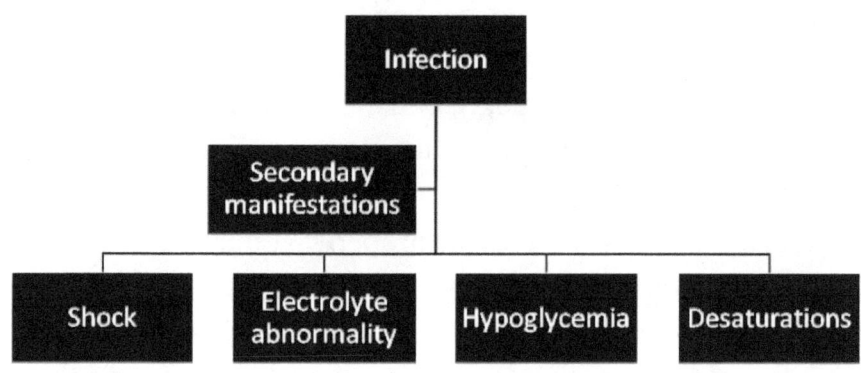

**Figure-1**   Primary cause and its cascade of secondary manifestations

One natural question that arises is why there was no seizures after admission even though the child was very sick. It is lucky that there were no seizures but baby was on the verge of throwing a seizure. Our actions were aggressive and we normalized all altered parameters very quickly so at the cellular levels everything went back to normal, so there was no seizure. We have aggressively corrected the shock, blood acidosis and hypoglycemia, there actions prevented the baby from seizures. For seizure to occur there should be prolonged energy failure, accumulation of excitatory amino acid glutamate externally, or there should be physical injury.

Why was baby not intubated on admission? This is because of my experience that, if you do certain things appropriately the baby won't need intubations and moreover I am confident of doing intubation in less than 30 seconds without fail. After blood parameter improvement baby's condition also improved, once baby's condition improves, he or she is unlikely to through a convulsion. Seizures are not random events but they are produced when cells are pushed into extremes of energy deficiency (shock, hypoglycemia, hypoxia) or electrolyte abnormalities.

Another question is why was inotropes given for such a long time when NIBP was absolutely normal after 6 to 12 hours. This is because of the difference in approach towards shock. For me shock is not just NIBP abnormality, it is the perfusion to the individual cells that matters. My definition of full control of shock is when there are no compensatory mechanisms working and there is no production of lactic acidosis. If there is lactic acid production beyond normal then that means some where there is anaerobic metabolism happening, some areas of body are under stress. As long as we are not in a position to pin point the cellular deficiency it is better to over treat shock rather than to under treat it. Shock was produced due the sepsis and till sepsis is not under full control subclinical shock can coexist. (read chapters on shock).

Why soda bicarbonate was given on admission even though it is an "untouchable" drug. According to my experience it is a wonder chemical if used judiciously. (Please read my chapter on shock and PALS). Actually, ventilation was avoided due to my use of soda bicarbonate. Body suffers most when the blood pH is abnormal, here with a pH of 7.108, cells are in the verge of collapse, and severe myocardial depression is also occurring, bodies buffering systems are exhausted, kidney takes long to restore this abnormality in this critical condition. So, we have to provide external help in the form of soda bicarbonate in a dilute form slowly along with normal saline push, it can harm nobody. Babies respiratory distress has multiple components, we have to split these into individual components and see, they are

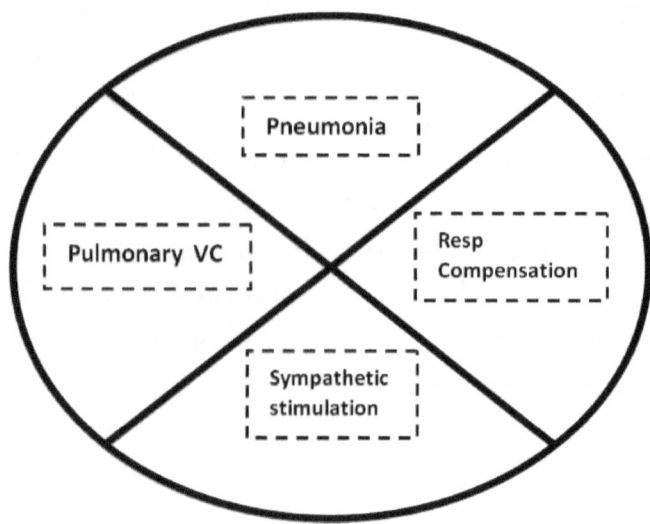

**Figure-2**  Respiratory distress due to different components

1. Respiratory distress component from pneumonia
2. Respiratory distress component due to pulmonary vasoconstrictions due to acidosis and hypoxemia.
3. Respiratory compensation component due to metabolic acidosis
4. Respiratory distress component due to sympathetic stimulation (anxiety and stress related, any living being on earth experiences utmost stress from near death like situation).

If you can tackle each of these components separately the individual effects on respiratory distress comes down. If you can treat the metabolic acidosis with soda bicarbonate and bring back the blood pH to > 7.3, the distress due to respiratory compensation goes away immediately and you can see the result, more over saturations improve because of the relaxation of pulmonary vasculature. (same principle is used in the use of soda bicarbonate infusion in PPHN).

Once saturations improve and distress comes down, your stress also goes away and now why on earth you should intubate?

In this case we have only done VBG not ABG, this is because we can get all the required results from VBG. It is easy to do and not painful and any staff can do this. Make it a habit of doing a VBG on admission for all babies, this can unravel several of the circulatory abnormalities. (also read chapter on VBG on admission…). whatever the disease you should have a bird's eye view of the problem, that mean you should know the primary cause, secondary and tertiary problems. You should know the chain of events and anticipate the next move of the disease. Never view each problem as an isolated event. For example, hypoglycemia occurring in a term child, treat the problem simultaneously search the events and causes leading to hypoglycemia.

## Chapter 16

# HOW CAN YOU EASILY TREAT BREATH HOLDING SPELLS (BHS)?

Breath holding spells are a common complaint seen in the OPD practice with varying intensity and frequency. Usually start presenting by 6 months of age but seen several cases before that age also. Some attacks are so dramatic and life threatening. Seen case with severe attacks requiring frequent mouth to mouth breathing for revival. Usual way of treating is reassurance, avoiding painful stimuli, prevent child from crying and starting on some iron preparation. But off late seen complete disappearance of breath holding spells with the use of vitamin D supplementations (adequately). I have experience in treating 10 to 15 cases of mild to severe BHS treated with iron and vitamin D. In this iron has only a small role to play because only after adding vitamin D in the regiment, I have seen dramatic response. The measured vitamin D levels invariably very low. Along with starting vitamin D rule out cardiac causes by doing an ECG and a 2D-Echo. Almost always 2D-Echo is normal.

> **Vitamin D alone in adequate doses can successfully treat most of the breath holding spells**

## MANAGEMENT OF BHS

Take detail history of presentation to differentiate between seizure and BHS

## BASIC INVESTIGATIONS

- Hb, Vitamin D, Ca, P
- ECG, 2D-ECHO
- ± EEG, MRI

## TREATMENT

- Iron supplementations
- Vitamin D in adequate doses (maintain vitamin D levels >50 nmol/L)
- Oral calcium supplementations
- In very severe, very frequent and life-threatening cases add anticonvulsant, best is Levetiracetam

**Seizure definition:** Seizure is a change in neurologic function (motor, sensory, experiential, or autonomic) that is associated with an abnormal synchronous discharge of cortical neurons.

From the behavior and applying the definition of seizures you can see breath holding spell is just a type of seizure. I have controlled most of my BHS cases with vitamin D and iron supplementation. One rare severe case (requiring several mouth-to-mouth resuscitations) as mentioned above was treated with levetiracetam and vitamin D, which responded well to treatment (EEG was normal as usual). After 6 months I was able to stop the anticonvulsant medications.

So, for all cases of BHS do vitamin D estimation and start on vitamin D supplementations along with iron supplementations. Maintain vitamin D levels above 40-60 ng/ml (100- 150 nmol/L).

## Chapter 17

# MANAGING A GASPING BABY REFERRED TO YOU (PLAYING GODS ROLE)

Receiving a gasping baby and reviving the baby is a challenge to any intensivist and there is nothing more satisfying than this. The number of these kind of cases has decreased over the decade with the availability of better transport facilities and better awareness and skill among doctors. Parental education also having a role to play. But in many less advanced states of India this can still be a real problem. These kind of transfers (gasping baby) usually occurs in the middle of night from sudden crashing of the baby, they come rushing without informing when consultants are least available. Whatever may be the case we have to revive the baby without much additional insults. Most babies reaching our NICU in gasping condition has survived without much added insults. If you recall the conditions on arrival the outcomes are excellent.

**CASE SCENARIO:**

A 5-day old FTND baby discharged home was brought to us from a nearby hospital in a gasping state with saturation non measurable, heart rate <30/minute, fully cyanosed, limp, in severe shock. Baby came crashing into the NICU at 11 am. How can you revive this baby without much further brain damage?

**IMMEDIATE MANAGEMENT**

Immediately give bag and mask ventilation with 100% oxygen, simultaneously start external cardiac massage. This will improve the heartrate and saturations, if required give IV adrenaline as usual dose, once HR improves >100/minute, SPO2 improves, intubate the baby immediately. Mobilize nursing teams, ask one team to prepare ventilator, another team for IV-line, long line and arterial line. Check glucose, if less than 60 mg/dl, give a push and start appropriate IVF. Sent a VBG immediately, start normal saline push with added soda bicarbonate,2ml/kg (higher dose may be needed here due to severe metabolic acidosis), give IV antibiotics, meropenem and amikacin / netilmicin within 30 minutes of admission and start vancomycin after finishing the initial infusion of antibiotics. Start inotropes, dopamine + dobutamine and adrenaline. Start inotropes in a higher dose of at least 16 to 20 mic/kg/minute (can start with lower dose in less severe cases and titrate). Maintain mean BP at a higher range. Sometimes inotropes rate needs to be increased up to 20-24 mic /kg/minute, increase the dose of adrenalin appropriately. In these critical situations it is better to start with a higher dose that increasing in small increments. If shock is not responding give a bolus and maintenance dose of hydrocortisone, here it was not given. Give Vitamin-k and H2 blocker to decrease the stress associated GIT hemorrhages. If there are any signs of seizures like tonic posturing or tonic-clonic convulsions start on Phenobarbitone and if required Fosphenytoin can be added. Connect to the ventilator once it is ready. Correct all the electrolyte abnormalities, give IV calcium gluconate and IM magnesium sulphate. Send all the investigation.

## Summary of actions taken in managing the gasping baby

- Bag and mask ventilation
- Intubation and connect to the ventilator
- IV adrenaline (as part of resuscitation)

- Normal saline push with added soda bicarbonate for faster normalization of metabolic acidosis, 1st aim is to bring blood pH above 7.25 then to >7.35
- IV antibiotics within 30 minutes of admission
- Inotropes: Dopamine, Dobutamine and adrenaline
- ± Hydrocortisone (not given in our case)
- IVF, inj. vitamin-K, IV ranitidine
- Correction of electrolyte abnormalities
- IV calcium gluconate + IM magnesium sulphate

One mistake doctor's make is put the baby on a less than adequate ventilatory settings. You have to put the baby on at least moderate to high settings when the baby is in a critical condition, means higher rate, high pressure, high $FIO_2$. This is to completely take over the respiration including respiratory compensatory component. Till the blood metabolic acidosis is corrected reasonably well we have to maintain respiratory compensation otherwise blood pH drops precipitously. Blood pH is the one which affects all the cellular function of the body, this is what every organism trying to defend vigorously. If we maintain on suboptimal settings baby may again slip into desaturations and respiratory failure sets in. It is very difficult to revive from frequent secondary deteriorations. This is because baby had collapsed and reached this state from exhaustion, so reviving baby from frequent deteriorations is not easy. Take x-ray chest with abdomen. Once baby is maintaining vitals on ventilator correct all the abnormal parameters one by one, completely analyze all the investigation reports and take action. Repeat blood gas, electrolytes and septic work up at regular intervals.

The following are the investigation report and the actions taken.

**Table: 1** Initial Investigation Reports, Interpretations & Actions taken

| Parameters | Results | Interpretations and actions to be taken |
|---|---|---|
| Birth weight | 3.2 kg | |
| Admission weight | 3 kg | Day-5 old, normal loss of weight |
| VBG | <table><tr><td></td><td>1st</td><td>2nd</td><td>3rd</td></tr><tr><td>pH</td><td>6.8</td><td>7.06</td><td>7.26</td></tr><tr><td>HCO3</td><td>4</td><td>9</td><td>14</td></tr><tr><td>BE</td><td>-28</td><td>-18</td><td>-10</td></tr><tr><td>PCO2</td><td>86</td><td>52</td><td>32</td></tr></table> | Severe metabolic acidosis and espiratory acidosis, sever base deficit, Ventilation with high setting and faster rate, give $NaHCO_3$ correction. |
| Hb | 10.5mg/dl, PCV 32 | Anemia/ Repeating Hb after 24 hrs. ± transfusion 15ml/kg to keep PCV > 40 |
| TC | 24,500 /P=86%/L=12%/E=2% | Increased, neutrophil predominance |
| Platelet | 89,000 /cu mm | Decreased, repeat after 24 hours |
| Urine RE | Pus cells: 10-15 pus cells HPF<br>RBC: 3-4 RBC/HPF | Urinary infection |
| GRBS | 78mg/dl | Normal |
| Na+ | 121 meq/L | Hyponatremia / needs correction |
| K+ | 6.2meq/L | Hyperkalemia / self corrects when acidosis is corrected, avoid K+ containing fluids |

| Parameters | Results | Interpretations and actions to be taken |
|---|---|---|
| iCa+ | 0.9 meq/L | Hypocalcemia / needs correction |
| Lactate | 88 mg/dl | Increased |
| SGOT | 152 IU/dl | Increased |
| SGPT | 88 IU/dl | Increased |
| Urea | 50 mg/dl | Mildly increased |
| Creatinine | 1.2 mg/dl | Mildly increased |
| CRP | 89mg/L | Increased |
| X-ray | B/L pneumonic patches | |

**Few points regarding blood gas correction:**

Blood pH is the factor which body is trying to defend vigorously. Body under normal conditions defend blood pH through respiratory and renal compensations. In critical condition like this it comes down only to respiratory compensation, in very critical states like near cardiac arrest renal compensation becomes irrelevant. In sepsis and shock, it is always metabolic acidosis and its respiratory system compensation which maintains blood pH. Once this respiratory compensation fails the pH nosedives and cardiac arrest ensures. This is what is happening for our baby. Its respiratory compensation part is important while reviving the baby. Once you put the baby on ventilator, don't straightaway discard the respiratory compensation part which baby was already doing by taking very deep breaths that too in a faster rate. So, while setting the ventilator, settings should be moderately high or high (depth and rate of ventilation). (You would have noticed sometimes after giving phenobarbitone, fentanyl etc. sudden deterioration in the form of desaturations can occur in a struggling respiratory distress baby, this is because of the sudden withdrawal of respiratory drive which was maintaining the saturations). Under ventilatory setting can result in crash, simultaneously if you correct metabolic acidosis part by giving diluted soda bicarbonate slowly the pressure on the system for compensation decreases and respiratory distress decreases. This is clinically shown as and called "synchronization with ventilator", "baby settling on ventilator" etc.

Intravenous soda bicarbonate helps in settling the baby very fast by faster normalization of metabolic acidosis. Even though soda bicarbonate is a "forbidden drug" for many, it is a very useful drug if used judiciously, knowing why we are using it. In severe metabolic acidosis body used all the reserve base excess (ie. $HCO_3^-$) for compensation, in that situation we should help the baby by providing soda bicarbonate externally what is wrong in that, here the argument that soda bicarbonate will be converted to carbon dioxide and worsens respiratory acidosis is a silly if you calculate the amount of carbon dioxide converted versus the carbon dioxide generated in the body. If respiratory acidosis is setting in then baby is in the exhaustion stage and need intubation for avoiding a crash in the near future. If babies respiratory drive is good (even with respiratory distress) then giving soda bicarbonate for metabolic acidosis correction is going to do wonders. That has multitude of effects like improvement of blood pH towards normal which improves all cellular enzymatic functions, prevent hyperkalemia, improves cardiac contractility etc.

**Three pillars of Management (PNM)**

- **Primary cause** correction
- **Normalization** of altered parameters
- **Maintenance** of normalized parameters

When this baby was brought to NICU, baby was on its way to cardiac arrest. Our first aim is to increase heart rate and saturation and correct shock as fast as possible. Most important factor for the baby is to maintain the blood pH in its normal range, baby was trying to maintain the blood pH by respiratory compensation, when that failed the blood pH dropped precipitously resulting in a crash. Our aim is to reveres everything in that order. Actions to be taken.

1. **Increase HR and saturations:** Bag & mask with 100% oxygen and ECM, intubate and connect to the ventilator.

2. **Correct metabolic acidosis and shock** – NS push + inotropes + soda bicarbonate

3. **IV antibiotics covering all organisms:** MDR G-ve, & MDR G+ve (MRSA, MRSE)

4. **Higher ventilatory setting (rate and depth)** – for respiratory wash out as part of respiratory compensation.

5. **Inj. vitamin K, IV ranitidine (stress GI bleeding prevention)**

6. **Correction of hypocalcemia** with IV calcium gluconate and magnesium sulphate IM

7. **Correction of hyponatremia:** calculate the amount and give ½ of that over 1 hour and the remaining over 24 hours, repeat the sodium after 6-8 hours.

8. **Hyperkalemia** gets corrected when metabolic acidosis is corrected, give IV calcium gluconate to counter the actions of hyperkalemia.

9. Do VBG or ABG regularly till blood pH is stabilized

10. Antibiotic policy should be dynamic according to the clinical condition and blood investigations reports, because infection is the primary insult here and that need to be hit

properly otherwise you are into trouble. (shock, TC, CRP, X-ray changes, oxygen requirements, etc.)

11. Packed cell transfusions, maintain PCV >40 %

12. Repeat septic workup and other investigations at regular intervals till they are normalized

The above-mentioned action has saved many lives in our NICU, the aggressiveness and the never give up attitude is one which helps us in achieving our goals. Don't aim for just survival of babies but aim for intact survival of babies. But there are many **pitfalls** (traps) which can lead to failures after the initial success.

**Pinfalls while managing a critical baby.**

- Inadequate treatment of **primary cause**, i.e. if sepsis overtakes, you are doomed for failure.
- Not taking care of **shock** properly, shock is the one which damages you baby's brain.
- Giving Inadequate **ventilatory** support.
- **Seizure**, if any should be aggressively managed.
- Not taking care of **altered parameters** – electrolytes, hypoglycemia, blood pH etc. If these are not taken care of then tertiary complications sets in like seizures from electrolyte abnormalities, cardiac arrythmias, brain damage from hypoglycemia etc. While analyzing altered parameters always ask yourself, how and why is it produced (root cause analyze).

If you fail to take care of any one of the above things then you are into trouble. We have to constantly keep a vigil on the primary cause (mostly it is infection) which led to secondary derangements. If the infection (primary cause) is not fully under control you are heading for a disaster, so, you should be ready to upgrade or add additional antibiotics without delay. Multiple resistant organisms would have entered into the baby, these can be MDR / PDR organisms or MRSA, unless you upgrade the antibiotics (based on the response) you are going to lose the baby. These kinds of very sick babies invariably have multiple types of organisms inside it as you upgrade antibiotics the sensitive once will get eliminated and the other resistant organisms will take over till you kill all. (always keep an open mind towards **multiple organ entry**). **Whenever a person is very weak commensals and colonizers from GIT, oropharyngeal mucosa can enter into the blood stream**. In normal condition also there is a constant streaming / seeding of organisms into the blood stream (fig.1). Usually, they gets eliminated by your immune system. This elimination is at default when you are in extreme stress.

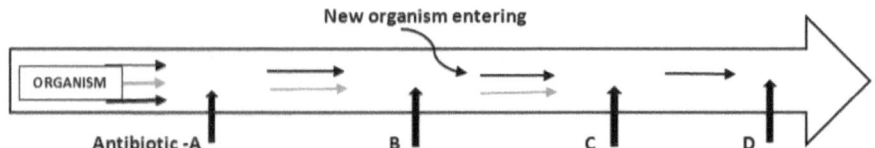

**Figure:1**    Multiple organ entry

The usual course is that baby survives the initial period only to deteriorate and die later. If you keep up your aggressive management and the vigil then you can see the success coming. From my experience the most important factors are control of infection and control of shock. In shock control your first aim is to bring up the mean BP to above normal. If you fail in bringing that very fast then you are going to lose the baby. Here is the step wise correction of shock.

1.  Normal saline pushes 20-30ml/kg ± added soda bicarbonate based on the blood gases.

2. Dopamine and dobutamine in moderately high or in high dose, don't waste time by increasing gradually. Don't decrease inotropes seeing high BP, these high BP are due to the release of counter regulating hormones (renin angiotensin aldosterone axis activation). If you start to decrease inotropes very early on seeing high BP then you are into a trap. Not a single baby had any problem related to hypertension over the years. Your first aim is to save the babe's life, all other things come only next.

3. If NIBP is not increasing even after 20 mic/kg/mt of dopamine and dobutamine combination, add adrenaline. In very much exhausted babies' adrenaline is very effective. When adding adrenaline never stop dopamine but can decrease the dose slightly but better do it after attaining stability. In case of refractory shock adrenaline and hydrocortisone can help.

4. If required give a bolus of hydrocortisone followed by maintenance doses.

5. The above steps should be very fast within half an hour. Assessment for response should be fast like reassessing every 5 to 10 minutes and 1/2 hourly.

6. Correct metabolic acidosis and sepsis, otherwise shock becomes resistant. Sometimes you can add 0.5 to 1 ml/hour of 1:1 diluted soda bicarbonate infusion to counter the continuous stream of metabolic acids produced, otherwise slow deterioration from blood pH fall can happen and end up in a crash if your nursing staff is not vigilant. For cells to function properly always keep blood pH above 7.3 and don't allow it to dip below that, if you allow it to dip then you are inviting trouble. If the dip happens myocardial depression happens and shock worsen and different levels of vicious cycles sets in. If metabolic acidosis is not getting corrected

that means shock is not getting corrected, all finger point towards uncontrolled infection.

7. If shock is not getting corrected change or add higher antibiotics, infection is the primary cause which created shock. Here at that critical period cultures are not going to help, you have to use your experience or you have to experiment, no textbook is going to lecture about this management. Textbooks or any lectures never discusses any life-threatening problems in depth, discussion never reaches that stage.

**Points to remember when ventilating a critical baby.**

1. Never under ventilate the baby, it produces stress on the baby, baby will be struggling to maintain parameters. Keep the respiratory compensation component working to keep the blood pH under control.

2. Setting should be atleast moderately high otherwise baby will be putting efforts, this is not good in the initial periods of a critical child. We have to take over the ventilation from the baby, not the other way around.

3. Assist control mode SIMV with higher support breaths will be the best mode of ventilation in the initial period.

4. Keep more than adequate FIO2 when there is shock, that increases dissolved oxygen delivery to the tissues.

5. Fully sedating the baby during the initial period is not good, as the babies respiratory drive goes away there can be difficulty in maintaining blood gas parameters. As and when everything is under control you can increase your sedation, surprisingly at this time sedation may not be required because once blood gases are settled baby also settles down. Baby's struggle is a struggle to maintain normal blood gases. There is a time lag between

equilibration of blood gases and the CSF fluid, so babies struggle can extend a bit longer than expected.

## Indicators of good control of sepsis and shock are,

1. Total count (TC) coming to normal (both leukopenia or leukocytosis returning towards normal)
2. Platelet counts improving towards normal
3. CRP and other inflammatory mediators decreasing
4. Most important one is shock coming under control. Even a trace of subtle shock indicates that shock is not fully under control. (subtle shock signs: poor color of baby, CRT 2-3 sec, increasing lactate, mild metabolic acidosis etc.)
5. Good urine output: usually a period of polyurea can be seen after good infection control. This is the retained interstitial fluid going out after control of infection. Also due to improvement in renal function. This is a good sign.
6. $SPO_2$ improving, oxygen requirement decreases.
7. GIT aspirate decreasing and becomes clearer. Signs of NEC improving.
8. Activity improving, a septic baby never has normal activity.
9. SGOT, SGPT normalizing
10. Hyponatremia improving
11. X-ray chest showing clearance
12. Overall color and appearance of the baby improving
13. Ventilatory setting improving.
14. Signs of PPHN going away
15. Seizures, apnea getting under control.

This much factors have to be considered before saying infection is under control. Don't just go by one factor like CRP or TC. When infection is under control means, the factors which has got deranged should all come to normal. Antibiotic resistance is rampant and is a reality in all ICU's worldwide, don't take an ostrich's attitude towards antibiotic resistant. Everybody may have seen many PAN drug resistant klebsiella, E-coli, Acinetobacter, Pseudomonas, MRSA etc. these may be inside your baby, how can you save the baby without killing them. If infection is not getting under control with the usual antibiotics you may have to consider giving the following groups of antibiotics.

1. Imipenem (better than meropenem because it is less used, less chance for resistance than meropenem, it is more costly so less widely used, more difficult to give than meropenem because of its precipitating nature)
2. For ESBL organisms – Tazobactam or Sulbactam combinations
3. Ciprofloxacin/Ofloxacin/ Levofloxacin
4. IV azithromycin, Clarithromycin (atypical organisms)
5. Colistimethate / Polymyxin-B (for PDR organisms)
6. Linezolid / teicoplanin / vancomycin / daptomycin (for MRSA, MRSE)
7. Tigicycline (for PDR organisms)
8. Sometimes need to add antifungals also based on C&S: fluconazole / amphotericin-B

**When are you justified in using extremely higher antibiotics?**

**In these extreme situations you are the only judge, nobody in this world can question you regarding your decision to use an antibiotic to save a life.**

- Any life-threatening situations where control of infection has not attained and any time delay would be life threatening for the baby. Also when culture report cannot be expected in the near future.

- Infection is not getting controlled and cultures are supporting a resistant organism.

- Whenever shock is not coming under control ever with adequate inotropic support you are justified in using higher antibiotics. (after ruling out noninfectious cause of shock)

- High suspicion of hospital acquired (ICU) infection. (Referred for another ICU or acquired from your own ICU).

- If you are confident that adding a higher antibiotic can save life then you are justified in using it. You are the only judge here and your conscience and experience should act here, others can only pray and criticize you from outside.

If you are adamant in not going for higher antibiotics because of your "protocols", then you are going to lose your baby only to blame on the fate. If you act smart, you can save a life - "taking over God's role". Protocols are never made for these extreme situations; they only cover the ordinary and common situations. MDR and PDR organisms are a reality, no point in taking an ostrich attitude.

What is the justification in changing an antibiotic based on cultures from superficial swabs like throat swab, GI aspirates, umbilical cord cultures or skin swab when blood cultures are sterile? This is a logical way of searching in the darkness. When you have nothing to guide and the baby is not improving you can use the list of colonized organisms as a guide for antibiotic policy. Baby gets colonized with organisms to whom it had contact with, these colonized organisms have more chance for entry into the blood stream. Whenever a baby falls sick these opportunistic colonized organisms enter the blood stream. So, rather than blindly choosing an antibiotic you can use the swab cultures as a guide. If the baby is doing well and everything is well under control there is no need for any change in antibiotics, unless you get a different blood culture positivity.

Over the decade I have managed dozens and dozens of gasping babies and am very confident in its management. I am not afraid of receiving a gasping baby. Because of this success I thought of sharing the subtle techniques with my readers. I know many of you are pioneers in this field and are managing many times better than me, still doctors not aware of the methods can use this in their practice. Let this book be an encouragement for expert clinicians to express their techniques through books. Journal publications are beyond reach of majority and lots of scrutiny knocks out the surprise element in it. Journals follow a predetermined path and no drastic innovations are allowed. Definitely doctors practicing outside are doing innovative ways of treatment and they are successful also.

Saving a gasping baby is like taking the role of God. Take this as a God given opportunity to save a life.

# Chapter 18

# SPEECH DELAY AND VITAMIN D DEFICIENCY

During our daily practice we come across several cases of delayed speech with no hearing defects. They may have a delay of 3 to 6 months or more when compared to peer groups. We know they will ultimately attain speech but this delay is worrisome for the parents. We should not miss a treatable cause; it is also worrisome for us. Over the years I have seen a strong association with prolonged vitamin D deficiency with speech delay. Now it is proved beyond doubt the usefulness of treating vitamin D deficiency in all cases of speech delay for getting a good response. I have been practicing this for more than 3 years.

## DELAY CAN BE IN THE FOLLOWING

1. Not specific words by 1-1/4 year of age
2. Not having 3 to 4 words vocabulary by 1-1/2 years
3. Not having 5 to 10 words and not joining 2 words by 2-1/2 years of age
4. Not joining 3 words by 3-1/2 years of age and very much reduced vocabulary.
5. Any parental concern for speech.
6. Less expressive speech and more sign language.

The above speech delay and any parental concern should prompt you to search for vitamin D deficiency. It is a known fact that hypothyroidism can also cause speech delay so, you should simultaneously rule out borderline hypothyroidism. So, do TSH,

Free T4, T4 and vitamin D. Speech delay is seen in children coming from gulf countries with nuclear families where one or both parents are employed and are living an apartment with no chance for sunlight exposure and social interactions. Features of autism are also more common in children from these families. This trend is fast catching up in our country because of the rapid urbanization and apartment culture and loss of joint family system. Invariably you can see a low level for vitamin D sometimes associated with borderline hypothyroidism. Any value of vitamin D <50 nmol/L* or <20ng/ml can be taken as abnormal (see table-1). But preferred levels are 40 to 60 ng/ml or 100 to 150 nmol/L

There is a catch in its interpretation, because many children due to speech delay may be on many vitamin supplementations, more over after coming from gulf (apartment life to village life) sunlight exposure may have improved and so the value of vitamin D can be near normal. This should not dissuade you from vitamin D treatment. It is the years of vitamin D delay which has manifested as speech delay. What are the steps to be taken?

1. Increase sunlight exposure, too early or too late slanting sunlight is not useful, UVB rays are needed.
2. Good social interaction of child and family members.
3. If age is appropriate send to playschool where interaction with kids gives a new lease of life.
4. Treat borderline hypothyroidism if it is present, always do TSH, T4, & free T4. Treat when TSH is >4 mIU/L and FT4 <1.2 ng/dl (sometimes can give a trial of thyroxine for 6 months with TSH values between 3.5 -4 mIU/L)
5. Treat with adequate amounts of vitamin D, I have seen treatment with inadequate doses for inadequate duration. Maintain vitamin D levels in the high normal range, 60 to

80 nmol/L. Daily doses with intermittent high bolus doses have shown the best response. Only bolus doses show partial response. Give weekly bolus doses initially for 3 to 4 months then can shift to fortnightly bolus doses. In very severe vitamin D deficiency cases with rickets, we usually give vitamin D as injections once in 2 to 3 months and seen excellent results.

   a. For 2-3 yr old I give vitamin D drops (800 IU/ml) 1.5 ml daily. Older children can use tab vitamin D available as 2000 IU strengths. Syrups only have 600 IU/5 ml in them, more recently one syrup with 2000 IU/5 ml has been introduced (Arachitol Nano 2000 IU/5ml).

   b. Drops Arachitol (60,000 IU/5ml): 2.5 ml weekly initially then fortnightly or use vitamin D sachet containing 60,000 IU per sachet.

   c. Or in severe cases injection vitamin D 6 lakh units IM once in 2 to 3 months, after 3 to 4 infections shift to oral preparations. Need to give daily doses for good response.

6. I usually don't send for speech therapy because the response is very quick and seen within weeks. Some severe older cases can be sent to speech therapist. Sending child to a playschool is a good speech therapy as other kids won't entertain sign languages and the urge for speech will be high, here kid teach kids how to speak.

7. I don't regularly check for vitamin D levels once treatment is initiated as the levels can be on the higher side (never in toxic range) and there is a tendency to stop it.

8. Never seen clinical signs of vitamin D toxicity. The vitamin D toxicity is over emphasized in literature. Now definition of vitamin D toxicity has been redefined, see table-1.

Of late we have seen several roles for vitamin D in the body, it is actually acting as a hormone. Of course, its actions are like thyroid hormones. Vitamin D like thyroid hormones are acting on the nuclear receptors almost activating one third of genes, that is phenomenal. It is some kind of facilitator in all cellular functions, it has role in rickets, developmental delay, speech delay, autism, immunity etc. See other chapters on vitamin D. Try this harmless form of treatment.

**Table:1**    (Royal Children's Hospital Melbourne guidelines)

| Classification | Vitamin D levels (nmol/L) | Vitamin D levels (ng/ml) |
|---|---|---|
| Severe deficiency | <12.5 nmol/L | <5 ng/ml |
| Moderate deficiency | 12.5 to 29 nmol/L | 5 to 11.6 ng/ml |
| Mild deficiency | 30 to 49 nmol/L | 12 to 19.6 ng/ml |
| Sufficient | ≥50 nmol/L | ≥20 ng/ml |
| Elevated | ≥250 nmol/L* | ≥100 ng/ml |
| Toxicity is defined as serum 25-OH-D >250 nmol/L (>100 ng/ml) with hypercalcemia and suppression of parathyroid hormone (PTH), PTH flattening happens at 30 ng/ml or 75 nmol/L range. | | |
| Preferred 25 (OH)D range is 40 to 60ng/ml or 100 to 250 nmol/L (Endocrinology society recommendation) | | |

# Chapter 19

# EARLY FEATURES OF AUTISM AND VITAMIN D DEFICIENCY

We can regularly see children coming with early features of autism in our OPD. The symptoms can vary from not interacting with the environment, mostly indulged in self-play, delayed speech, echolalia, poor eye to eye contact, living in their own world etc. These symptoms are more seen in children coming from gulf countries, flat dwellers and most are from nuclear families. There is less and less interaction with people and less exposure to the outside world and sunlight. The incidence of autism is increasing in proportion to the urbanization and collapse of joint family structure. More over excessive TV and mobile usage also contribute to the development of autism.

From observation over the years, I could draw a relationship of early autism with vitamin D deficiency from lack of sunlight exposure. I noticed this association for the past 5 years and treating early autism patients well. The response on well-established cases of autism is poor. There is a very good response once you start treatment with adequate amounts of vitamin D supplementation. Also make sure there is no associated borderline hypothyroidism, if present treat that with appropriate doses for sufficient duration. Approximately 25% of autistic children also have associated borderline hypothyroidism, 50% cases are detected based on the cut off value of free T4, in majority TSH values are normal. The response to vitamin D is good if you start treatment early and good response is seen in children below 3 years of age. For children below 2 years the response is excellent. As the age of the patient goes up the quickness of response comes down.

Also do thyroid screening at regular intervals. Very advanced and severe autism needs specialist level treatment with strict protocols.

Most children with autistic features are on multiple vitamin supplementations including that containing vitamin D, so value of vitamin D may be normal in that instant. This should not dissuade you from starting vitamin D supplements.

**BASIC INVESTIGATIONS:**

1. Hemoglobin
2. Vitamin D, Ca+, P
3. TSH, freeT4, T4

I am not going into the intricate classification of autism, whether my patients fit into autism spectrum disorders or not, more worried with the parental concern of autism. If able to rectify that concern, I am more than satisfied. Small features of autism if treated early can prevent autism in majority of cases. Advanced cases show resistance to treatment. Definitely the response is poor once autism is fully established. Some children with autistic features with intermittent aggressiveness also responds well to this simple treatment.

Most of my babies with features of autism have very low levels of vitamin D. Even if the spot vitamin D levels are near normal, they may have prolonged low levels over the years. Sometimes recent vitamin supplementation or sunlight exposure would have brought the vitamin D values to near normal. Most babies also have features of rickets like, leg bend, chest wall deformity, delayed closing of AF, or wide AF etc. Regarding borderline hypothyroidism TSH may show borderline elevation above 4, or free T4 shows low levels. Fifty percentage of time it is the low free T4 levels which prompt treatment. A Free T4 value of <1.2 ng/dl is taken as abnormal for babies having development delay or features of autism, TSH cut off is lowered further than 4 to even up to 3.5 to get the benefit of doubt to the children. These babies are given a trial of Thyroxine for 6 months, if response is good thyroxine treatment is continued). I want to give the benefit of doubt to the child rather than risk development delay. Over the decade TSH cut off value is coming down from 10 to the current level and we don't know where it is heading!

I have seen several 2-3 year-old kids coming with development delay after consulting from reputed hospitals, bringing along with them reports of abnormal thyroid screening values. They have overlooked several of these borderline values. (TSH 4.15, 4.75, 5 etc.). These borderline cases responded well to treatment. These babies also had low vitamin D levels. Whenever a case of autism comes rule out hypothyroidism and start treatment with vitamin D in adequate dose and duration. Definitely your children improve.

God has created the universe and supplied vitamin D in abundance through sunlight. Since sunlight is freely available 12 hours a day did not stuff other food items with vitamin D. But we people prove it all wrong by not getting into sunlight and deficiency spreaded like wild fire, slowly recognizing its role. Recent increased spurt in several diseases like cancer, autism, infertility, hypothyroidism, developmental delay, etc. all can have a role in vitamin D deficiency. Needs thorough investigations. Covid-19 pandemic is worst in western world and in urban cities where there is lack of sunlight exposure. There is a definite role for vitamin D in immunity.

## Chapter 20

# DEVELOPMENT DELAY OR LAG AND VITAMIN D DEFICIENCY

In our OPD practice we come across several cases of development lag or delay without any significant cause in the perinatal period, mostly presenting under the age of 3 years. Sometimes they may improve over the months but is a huge worry for the mother and doctor. Never dismiss this as normal and wait for the catching up to occur naturally. Doctors usually reassure them or do a thyroid screening. Over the years we have come across a definite cause for this delay, it is due to the **prolonged Vitamin D deficiency**. Due to the decreased sunlight exposure over the decades, there is severe vitamin D deficiency in the mother and the baby, several babies are born with features of rickets (very wide AF, soft skull bones, deformed chest etc.). Simultaneously make sure that there is no associated borderline hypothyroidism. If you start treatment with "adequate dose" (here adequate dose is on the higher side) within weeks you can see the mother saying with a smile on her face that her baby has started attaining milestones. This is what we want from our baby, to attain milestones at regular intervals. This discovery was a very satisfying that we could treat most if not all of the development delay coming to our OPD. This we want to share with the world and can do more studies on these.

If we screen our babies with the development charts available, there is a big gap confidence interval [ $3^{rd}$ to $97^{th}$ percentile] for each mile stones, this is actually delaying the investigations. If we are applying this as a guide, we will not take any actions immediately as the child has more time to attain that particular mile stone. For example, according to TDSC chart (Trivandrum Developmental Screening Chart) the confidence interval for rolling back to stomach is from 4 months of age to 12 months of age, for self to sitting position is from 7.5 months to 13 months, for walks with help is from 10.5 months to 17.5 months, walks alone is 11.5 months to 20 months, these are some of the examples and these are too wide to follow practically. Should my baby wait this long before any action is taken? My suggestion is to take the 50th centile as the cut off for taking basic actions (vitamin D and thyroid screening). A screening test should be able to pick up the altered growth at its slightest deviation from normal.

My child's potential may be better than the laggards of general population. It is better to stick on with the 50th centile. Every mother wants their baby to grow according to their growth potential so, don't deny their child this simple way for improvement. Whenever you see a baby with slightest of delay or any parental concern of delay check the following.

**Table:1**  Basic Investigations for all Development delay or lag in Children.

| Investigations | Cut off | Treatment |
| --- | --- | --- |
| Vitamin D | Normal range 20 to 100 ng/ml or 50 to 250 nmol/L  Preferred range: 40 to 60 ng/ml or 100 to 150 nmol/L | Daily adequate dose + Intermittent bolus doses |
| TSH | >4 IU/ml start treatment  (some borderline cases of TSH >3.75 IU/ml can give a trial of treatment, if no response from vitamin D therapy alone) | Give treatment for at least up to 3 years of age or at least for 2 years whichever is later.  Trial of treatment for 6 months and see the response, if good response continue treatment. |

| Investigations | Cut off | Treatment |
| --- | --- | --- |
| Free T4 | Treat all symptomatic cases with free T4 values below 1.2 ng/dl. | Give benefit of doubt to the already compromised patient. Exact ideal values are still a distant dream. |
| T4 | See specific cutoffs | |

With this treatment strategy most of the cases of developmental delay can be improved. This strategy can also be applied to known cases of cerebral palsy / development delay also, because we have seen definite improvements with vitamin D and correction of borderline hypothyroidism. Most of the CP children are vitamin D deficient from lack of sunlight exposure. All known cases of developmental delay and CP patients should be screened for hypothyroidism and vitamin D deficiency. Our aim should be to prevent additional insults creeping up.

## TREATMENT OF VITAMIN D DEFICIENCY

Aim is to maintain a higher vitamin D level in blood, >50 nmol/L (60 to 80 nmol/L), from experience it is seen that best response is seen with daily supplementations with intermittent large bolus doses weekly or fortnightly depending on the severity. Values around 30 nmol/L (recommended normal level) (see table-2) will not consistently produce the desired results. The response is not uniform with large bolus dose of vitamin D from sachets or capsules (60,000 IU/sachet or capsule). For severe rickets with severe chest deformity and severely bowed legs the best response is with injection vitamin D IM once in 2-3 months with daily supplementations of vitamin D with added calcium. So, for the developmental delay we can follow the following regimen.

1. Daily vitamin D 800 to 2000 IU per day of vitamin D depending on the age and weight.

2. Give bolus of Vitamin D sachets or syrup solutions containing 60,000 IU/5ml, give in a dose of 1.5 ml/ 2ml /2,5ml / 3 ml weekly initially then once in 2 weeks till full recovery. For severe developmental delay given injection vitamin D and seen good response.

3. It is better to supplement with calcium, as the calcium requirement increases once you start vitamin D supplementation. Calcium assimilation into bone increases many folds once you start vitamin D supplementation.

4. Once good recovery is attained you can maintain on vitamin D supplementation alone.

5. Encourage daily sunlight exposure (9 am to 4 pm) (UVB rays). Very early and late evening sunlight (very slanting sunlight) is not very useful. There are no recommended exposure times but 10 to 15 minutes seems sufficient.

6. I don't encourage repeated vitamin D estimation if you are taking bolus dose of vitamin D as the levels can be high and will be forced to stop supplementations and your higher goal of treatment of development delay will remain a distant dream. If you are particular in doing vitamin D estimation you have to time this with bolus dose, just prior to the next bolus dose will be a good strategy to know the trough value.

7. Duration of treatment is common sense as on stoppage of vitamin D supplementation the level goes to below normal. Correction of neurologic deficit is a long-drawn process, brain may be doing the repair work of altered / defective or deficient neuronal circuitry, neurotransmitter changes etc. So

prolonged supplementation is suggested, after all it is just a vitamin supplementation whose exact role is still a mystery.

**Table: 2** (Royal Children's Hospital Melbourne Guidelines)

| Classification | Vitamin D levels (nmol/L) | Vitamin D levels (ng/ml) |
|---|---|---|
| Severe deficiency | <12.5 nmol/L | <5 ng/ml |
| Moderate deficiency | 12.5 to 29 nmol/L | 5 to 11.6 ng/ml |
| Mild deficiency | 30 to 49 nmol/L | 12 to 19.6 ng/ml |
| Sufficient | ≥50 nmol/L | ≥20 ng/ml |
| Elevated | ≥250 nmol/L* | ≥100 ng/ml |
| Toxicity is defined as serum 25-OH-D >250 nmol/L (>100 ng/ml) with hypercalcemia and suppression of parathyroid hormone (PTH), PTH flattening happens at 30 ng/ml or 75 nmol/L range. | | |
| Preferred 25 (OH)D range is 40 to 60ng/ml or 100 to 250 nmol/L (Endocrinology society Recommendation) | | |

## DISCUSSION

For most babies with development delay, the perinatal history and brain MRI scans are absolutely normal. Delay can be gross motor, fine motor or in language. They can also show tonal abnormalities. Usually, if left alone they will catch up over the years, but sometimes with permanent delay. If you allow for natural catch up to occur, these babies will definite loose some of its developmental potentials which is very difficult to measure. Vitamin D, through its actions through nuclear receptors, activate thousands of genes and have definite role in the growth of central nervous system circuitry. Thyroid hormones also act through nuclear receptors, all cells have these receptors. Over the years we have not yet discovered the exact roles in the CNS development process. These acts as facilitatory hormones which are giving continuous signals on a daily basis to the cells. If they are deficient all the fundamental architecture of the brain gets altered, including myelinations, synaptic connections, synaptic signaling, oligodendrocyte functions, microglial growth etc. we are actually searching for a black cat in a dark room, intense research is needed to unveil the mysteries behind vitamin D. for the present movement what we can do is screen and supplement and make a routine for sunlight exposure. Over the years there is gradual decline in the amount of sunlight exposure for the population in general due to the increasing urbanization and apartment residential culture.

In summary whenever you see a child with developmental lag or delay start vitamin D in sufficient quantity and duration. Simultaneously rule out there is no associated borderline hypothyroidism, while doing that always do TSH and freeT4. Keep TSH cut off low (3.5 to 4-IU/ml) and freeT4 cut off high 1.2ng/dl for children below 3 years of age as their brain is still in a faster growing phase. In this chapter I have not discussed the metabolic causes leading to developmental delay, which any standard textbook can give.

**"let's allow the sun to shine over our head for a brighter future"**

## Chapter 21

# AN OVERVIEW OF MECHANISMS OF DEVELOPMENT DELAY

To understand the mechanisms for developmental delay it is easy if we understand the normal development process occurring in the brain. I am not going into embryology part, but gives an overview of the process. Baby's growth from a fertilized ovum to a complex human being is a well-orchestrated ballet and all the required instructions are engraved in its genome. It is well programmed and self-sufficient that all the needed commands, checks and balances are inside the genome. Basically, the brain development can be summarized through the following steps. Brain growth involves neurogenesis (neuron multiplication), neuronal migration, neural and glial cell differentiation, myelination, synaptogenesis, development of nuclei (aggregation of neurons to execute a specified function), development of hierarchical control of different parts of brain, memory etc.

After fertilization, the permutations and combination of genes for that individual is fixed. The individual then develops according to the signal engrained in it. If there are chromosomal defects, then the sequence of events controlled by that missed chromosome is disrupted. If there are no defects, then the journey is smooth. This journey becomes rough when insults occur on its pathway. Insults can be in different forms and will discuss later. The brain develops from ectodermal layer and see any embryology text for elaborate details.

- **Neurogenesis:** in this the cells bordering the ventricles and ducts differentiate (germinal matrix) to become neurons and they multiply in numbers. Any insult in this stage cause exponential decrease in final number of neurons, results in microcephaly and severe brain impairments.

- **Neuronal migration:** the neuronal cells bordering the ventricles after multiplication migrate to the different parts of the brain through predetermined pathways. This is called neuronal migration, any disruption in this stage has huge consequences. Insult can be in the form of infections, ischemia, hemorrhage, toxic metabolites, hypoxemia, hypoglycemia etc.

- **Neural and glial cell multiplication and differentiation:** neurons after reaching their destination continuously multiply to reach the required number of neurons. These neurons also undergo differentiation. The glial cells are the supporting cells for neurons. It supports its growth by providing nutrition, supports physically, creates a supportive microenvironment, may also provide signals for multiplication and growth.

- **Myelination and synaptogenesis:** these are an ongoing process; mature neurons develop myelin sheath essential for its function. Millions and millions of synaptic connections are made, quality and quantity of these make a person average, above average or brilliant. This can be seen in one person's quality of action, quality of thinking, quality of physical movements, skills etc.

- **Development of nuclei:** nuclei are aggregates of neurons with a common function. Complex circuits are formed internally and develops connections tracts with other centers. This is an ongoing process.

After birth, brain growth won't stop all of a sudden but continues at a rapid pace. This can be seen indirectly as a rapid increase in head circumference. HC increases by 12 cm in the first year, 6 cm in the second year. In the first 7-9 months of life, 70 percentage of brain growth of an adult is completed and within 2 years 90 percentage of growth is over and by first 3 years nearly 95% of brain growth is complete. So, the first 3 years of life is the most important period in an individual's life. Interventions can work wonders during this period, similarly any insults during this period can run havoc. During the initial newborn period neurons retains the ability to multiply, after that this ability is lost. Myelinization of brain is nearly complete in the first 3 years of life.

A concept call **brain plasticity** works during the first 3 years of life. During brain development lots of construction and destructive events (remodeling) are happening simultaneously. Using plasticity of brain, the neurons or areas meant for destruction can be saved and utilized for better purposes. By utilizing plasticity, we can save these areas from destruction and instead use these areas as an alternative for area already destroyed. Early intervention (physiotherapy) has a major role in utilization of plasticity of brain. Area mend for destruction can be diverted for better purpose. This ability of plasticity is not seen in mature brain.

**Various mechanisms of brain damage or brain growth faltering.**

1. Inherent genetic abnormality in the form of chromosomal anomalies like aneuploidy, inversion, deletion, microdeletions, long repeats, single gene defect etc.
2. Inborn errors of metabolism (IEM)
3. Intra uterine TORCH infections.
4. Hypoxic Ischemic Encephalopathy (HIE), perinatal insults.
5. Sepsis and shock
6. Infectious insults like meningitis, brain abscess.
7. Hormonal and other deficiencies like hypothyroidism, vitamin-D deficiency.

8. Damage from hypoglycemia and electrolyte abnormalities
9. Brain insults due to clinical and non-clinical seizures (EEG seizure).
10. Lack of environmental stimulation
11. Severe PEM and growth faltering.
12. Stroke / infarct/ cerebral edema
13. Maternal diseases causing brain growth faltering.

In summary these can be grouped under the following categories.

- **Defective growth potential** of brain from the beginning (genetic defects group)
- **Acquired one-point insults** on a genetically normal brain (HIE, Stroke, infections,)
- **Ongoing insults** on normal brain or abnormal brain (hypothyroidism, vitamin D deficiency, lack of stimulation, recurrent seizure, IEM)

## DEFECTIVE GROWTH POTENTIAL

In this category due to genetic defect there is inherent defect in the growth potential. But can be utilize whatever growth potential is there through early intervention strategies. Make sure no added insults occur on its pathway through regular screening for hypothyroidism and vitamin D deficiency. Additional insults like seizures, lack of environmental stimulations, other nutritional deficiencies should be tackled appropriately.

## ACQUIRED ONE POINT INSULT

In this one-point insult category (HIE, stroke, infections) also the above-mentioned points hold good. Depending of the age of insult the effectiveness of plasticity of brain can vary, utilize this early intervention strategies to the maximum. Beware of the added insults like hypothyroidism, vitamin D deficiency propping up.

## ONGOING INSULT

Ongoing insults on normal or abnormal brain can cause further deteriorations. Ongoing insults can be hypothyroidism, vitamin D deficiency, recurrent clinical or subclinical seizures (EEG abnormality alone) should be tackled efficiently. Each insult has its own contributions towards damage. If everything is taken care off, we can get maximum out of the child.

# Chapter 22

# PITFALLS IN THE MANAGEMENT OF DEVELOPMENTAL DELAY

**(Never miss a case of borderline hypothyroidism or vitamin D deficiency)**

I am saddened by the masterly inactivity attitude shown by many doctors towards a child with development lag or delay. Have seen dozens and dozens of cases of developmental delay where simple investigations would have unravelled the cause of delay. But opted for masterly inactivity and precious time is lost in the process. Development delayed child will attain milestones one by one at a slow pace and don't glorify the slowly attained milestones, don't delay simple investigations.

## INTRODUCTION

Developmental delay happening to a child is the most traumatizing experiences for parents. Parents always ask, is my child going to be ok. This is a very difficult question for a paediatrician to answer. But with existing evidence we are bound to give a reasonable answer. Developmental delay is a practitioner's nightmare as under ordinary set up it acts as a dead end. Most doctors look for higher centre's prescription for clues, and they stop thinking once they had found out one diagnosis like cerebral palsy or an incident in the new born period for blaming for the delay. (for example, like h/o HIE, meconium aspiration, ventilation in the newborn period or just extended NICU stays). A child labelled CP is a lifelong label. Even if you label a child with CP, there can be ongoing additional insults happening over and above the static insult already received. After the initial insult brain is constantly remodelling itself with the available resources. If you can provide a good environment through early intervention strategies brain can show tremendous catch up. Any ongoing insults should be screened at regular intervals. At least some doctors are missing these ongoing insults like borderline hypothyroidism and vitamin-D deficiency. (according to my experience vitamin D has a huge role to play in brain development, discussed in detail later and in other chapters) Due to brain plasticity we can constantly remodel the brain through early intervention strategies.

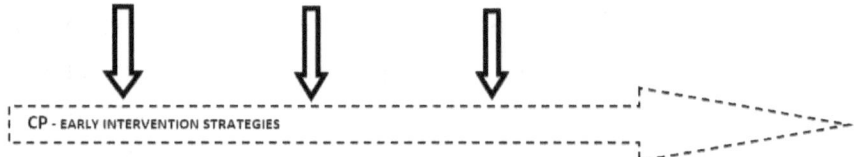

**Figure:1** Developing brain and ongoing insults

## Let us look into factors relating to developmental delay and where are we making mistakes?

Development of a child from embryo to a full human being is a miracle. Brain is composed of billions and billions of cells and have trillions and trillions of synaptic connections. Development from embryo to an adult is a well-orchestrated miracle. Any decrease in number of cells or decrease in number of synaptic connections or any deviations in neuronal connections (migration defects) can have longstanding impact on intellect and memory which is not exactly measurable. Brain growth and its evolution is ultra-complex and incomprehensible. Brain growth involves neurogenesis, neuronal migration, neuronal and glial cell differentiation, myelination and synaptogenesis. Then there is acquisition of different functions by neurons or groups of neurons (called nuclei), and their coordination and control by higher centres, voluntary control, memory etc. These complicated developmental processes are under genetic, hormonal (chemical) and environmental control. The insult occurring at different phases has different effects with respect to the degree of damage and qualitative defects.

## Brain damage can occur in any of the following ways from the embryo period to adulthood.

- Genetic abnormality causing derangement of normal pattern of development, these include chromosomal abnormalities (eg: downs syndrome), single gene defects, inborn errors of metabolism (IEM) etc. Nothing much can be done in this. But treat any additional insults happening, like hypothyroidism, uncontrolled seizure occurring during development, so always screen for these at regular intervals. Early intervention can modify their evolution.

- Intrauterine infections causing quantitative and qualitative damage to neurons and supporting cells. (eg. TORCH infections resulting in microcephaly and developmental delay)

- Ischemic insult resulting in neuronal loss (HIE, shock, stroke etc)

- Hypoglycaemia, hyperbilirubinemia induced neuronal damage.

- Recurrent or prolonged seizure induced damage.

- Postnatal infection induced damage. (eg. sepsis, meningitis)

- Delayed brain development from lack of gene signalling for development, like for example as in hypothyroidism, vitamin –D deficiency.

- Lack of environmental stimulation as that occurring for children in care homes, children with neglected parents, etc.

- Severe nutritional deficiencies.

Developmental delay (divided into 3 major groups for convenience)

- **Relatively** untreatable group, like chromosomal anomalies, IEM, brain damage from one point insult like HIE. (Even though insults are untreatable but modifiable through early interventions). Here also always look for treatable causes creeping up at regular intervals for example, hypothyroidism, vitamin-D deficiency. This relatively untreatable group also shows fair improvement if given proper early intervention measures starting from an early stage, preferably from NICU itself.

- **Treatable group with obvious causes** like hypothyroidism with definite cut off values. (for eg. like TSH value > 4 IU/ml or free T4 values <1.2ng/ml)

- **Treatable but missed group:** In this group there are conditions which can be missed by many doctors. These are children with subclinical or borderline hypothyroidism, vitamin D deficiency induced developmental delay, language delays etc.

Developmental delay is a commonly encountered entity by practicing doctors with high degree of mismanagement. It is very painful to see a child being mismanaged by lack of awareness on part of a treating doctor. There are several causes for developmental delay, most are less responsive to treatment but never miss a simple treatable cause like hypothyroidism, vitamin D deficiency. It amounts to negligence if you miss a case of hypothyroidism in a developmental delay baby. The screening for hypothyroidism done at birth is not an excuse for missing hypothyroidism later. Any time developmental delay later is an excuse for doing thyroid screening, I also do vitamin D estimations. There are several causes for missing developmental delay, which will be discussed later. Once the growing age is over measuring developmental delay becomes more and more difficult like for example if the child has passed 3 years of age then there are less measurable milestones. Then intelligence, memory, physical skills etc comes into play and these are not properly measurable and comparable, it has wide variation among children. Any growth faltering noticed by parents or other practitioner should be taken seriously. I have observed several doctors not taking seriously the parental concern of growth delay and missing the golden opportunity for intervention. For example, mother saying my child has not started standing up with support by one year of age and doctor reassuring it as normal is not proper. If you are reassuring the mother, please make sure to follow up this child after one or two months and look for catch up. If there is no catch up definitely rule out hypothyroidism and vitamin D deficiency as a cause for delay.

Development charts for screening purpose can be misleading, as the time gap allowed for each milestone is huge, any average child's growth should follow at least $50^{th}$ percentile line for the general population, if he or she is not following that do investigations to rule out hypothyroidism or vitamin D deficiency

Please remember the following in developmental delay,

- Corrected age: calculate development based on corrected age for preterm babies.
- Take action when there is slippage of development by the next milestone.

**Table:1**   Milestones and Usual Appearing Age

| Milestones | Usual milestone appearing age | Practical cut off limit to act |
|---|---|---|
| Social smile | Must appear within 2 months of age | Take action if no social smile by 2 months of age, or if quality of smile is not up to the mark. |
| Supine to prone | By 4 months of age | Take action if baby has not rolled over by 6 months |

| Milestones | Usual milestone appearing age | Practical cut off limit to act |
|---|---|---|
| Head control | By 6 months of age | Take action if no head control by 6 months |
| Kneeling | By 8 months | Take action if not kneeling by 9 months |
| Sitting | By 9 months | Take action if not sitting by 11 months |
| Standing with support | By 11 months | Take action If not standing with support by 1 year |
| Independent walking | By 1 year | Take action if not walking few steps independently by 1 year & 2 months. |
| Speech | Few words by 1 year | No words by 1 year 2 months take action/ any parental concern take action |
| | By 1-1/2 year should have 5-8 words | Take action if there are no words or if parents are concerned. |
| | By 2 years should have 8-15 words, should join 2 words | By 2-1/2yrs if that is not there take action / any parental concern take action |
| Parental concern of mile stones | | Take action whenever there is parental concern on milestones. |
| Look for autistic features or tendencies for that | Self-play, no proper eye to eye contact, less social interaction, severe expressive language delay, abnormal repetitive action, excessive hand regard etc. | Start investigation |

- Take due concern when mother says my child is not performing when compared to other sibling or any other child of his or her age. These may be the first hinds of developmental delay. Don't miss these as mother may not tell you a second time when she notices a delay because of shyness or because of your reassurance. Always ask for history of prematurity.

- When using TDSC chart some milestones are miles long (confidence intervals are too wide) like for example supine to prone, walk with help, raising self to sitting position etc. TDSC chart are made for screening purpose, your baby in front of you have passed the screening stage and you should not miss treatable causes any further. You can use $50^{th}$ percentile values as cut off for screening. You are dealing with a child who is already suspected for developmental delay. You should not take cut off at $3^{rd}$ percentile for the general population for your child, this results in undue delay in taking actions. Don't place your child in the non-performers category by comparing with groups in the $3^{rd}$ centile line.

- Always ask for details of early interventions undergone. Needs to undergo physiotherapy only under properly trained physiotherapist. No need to start physiotherapy if there is only a developmental lag and see for the response from other interventions. Definitely start if the developmental lag or delay is associated with tonal abnormalities, tight angles or abnormal reflexes. Undergoing physiotherapy under untrained physiotherapist is like not doing anything at all or is like doing some passive flexion and extension exercise. So, doctors must be vigilant while referring a baby for OT-PT, always refer to a properly trained paediatric physiotherapist. If you are not seeing the desired result from physiotherapy don't be hesitant in changing the physiotherapist.

From my 15 years of experience apart from definite cases of CP and diagnosed cases of development delay, other major groups of developmental delay are due to overt hypothyroidism, subclinical hypothyroidism and vitamin D deficiency. Treating these problems shows definite improvement in the next visit itself. My yard stick for improvement is my examination findings, mother's words and mother's happy face of her child attaining next milestone. During my early years of practice only treatable cause was overt hypothyroidism and lots of babies failed to show any improvement and I was really asking "am I missing anything". That question led to the finding that, lots of babies were showing low vitamin D levels and also notices borderline values for TSH and free T4. Treating with vitamin D and borderline cases of hypothyroidism over these years showed great improvement for my babies. Gradually I could make out the clinical cut off values where we can get optimal growth for our babies. For TSH cut off was kept at >4mIU/ml and all babies are given vitamin D. (almost most babies had low levels of vitamin D). Still further borderline values of TSH (3.5 to 4 IU/ml) with definite developmental delay was given a trial of thyroxine for 6 months, and continued with that if these babies are showing catch up growth. This is because you want to get maximum outcome from your babies as you are in the golden period of brain development (1st 3 years of life). I don't want to miss this opportunity. Sixty to seventy percent of babies showed very satisfactory improvement (good response), another 20 percent showed slow but satisfactory improvement and the rest (20%) showed no improvement.

Another funny thing noticed over these years was that the cut off for TSH was coming down from >10 mIU/ml to approximately 4 to 5 today. Why did that happen over the 15 years period, with this high TSH cut off we have denied treatment and better quality of life for millions and millions of children, what is the economic cost for the society, whom to blame? My understanding is that we are still in the nascent stage of understanding the human physiology. So, cut offs are not the last word and it is the clinical response that matters. Cut offs keeps on changing until we understand human physiology fully. So, by giving a trial of thyroxine for borderline cases of hypothyroidism you are not going to harm the child and if you are seeing a good response continue thyroxine or otherwise stop it.

- Definite hypothyroidism: TSH >4 mIU/L or free T4 <1.1 ng/dl
- Borderline hypothyroidism: TSH 3.5 to 4 mIU/L, free T4 values between 1.1 - 1.2 ng/dl
- Keep Vitamin D (25-OH-D) levels above >40 ng/ml or >100 nmol/L **(preferred range: 40 to 60 ng/ml or 100 to 150 nmol/L)**
- Vitamin D toxicity 25-OH-D >100 ng/ml or 250 nmol/L with hypercalcemia and suppression of parathormone (PTH)

**For developmental delay do the following investigations (list is incomplete)**

First level screening test for all babies showing developmental delay:

1. Haemoglobin
2. TSH, Free T4, T4, T3
3. Vitamin D
4. Alkaline phosphatase, Calcium, Phosphorous,
5. SGOT, SGPT
6. Urea, creatinine, $Na^+$, $K^+$

   For selected subgroup of babies, or babies not showing improvement

7. MRI

8. EEG (if seizures or suspicion)

9. Karyotyping if any dysmorphism

10. Metabolic screening (if any suspicion)

11. FISH, tests for deletion, inversion etc according to the suspicion.

Treatment strategies for developmental delay

1. Treat the deficiency properly (never to undertreat deficiencies, even if you slightly over treat the deficiencies it is going to be ok.)

2. If values are borderline be bold enough to give a trial for 6 months.

3. Always give vitamin D for all cases of development delay in adequate doses for adequate duration.

4. Start Intensive early intervention for needy babies.

5. Regular follow up.

In the case of thyroid screening almost 50 % of hypothyroid cases are found from low values of free T4. Most of the doctors don't look into free T4 values. For TSH keep a low cut off for babies showing developmental delay or lag. TSH cut off is kept at 4 mIU/L. For babies showing developmental delay and with thyroid values between 3.5 mIU/L and 4 mIU/L give a trial of thyroxine for 6 months and see the results, if response is good continue with treatment. This is for giving the benefit of doubt to the baby who is already compromised. I have painfully seen development delay babies coming after consultation from premier institutes with TSH values of 4.7 mIU/L, 5.2 mIU/L and not being treated. They have either overlooked these results or they are following a higher cut off. These children show excellent improvement after starting thyroxine. Only sorry for the lost time. **(TSH, mIU/L =IU/ml)**.

When we were undergraduates the TSH cut off for treatment was >10 IU/ml, (1997) over the years the cut off is coming down, there is more probability for it to come down further to values near 2.5 IU/ml. This has causes treatment denial for millions and millions of babies, whom to blame for this, we doctors are blindly following these recommendations. This is the reason for me to dig my own path in my cases of both vitamin D and borderline hypothyroidism.

Most CP babies invariably be inside homes and so have very low vitamin-D values because of lack of sun exposure. They show improvement once we start vitamin D in the form of changes in tonal abnormalities, better social interaction, improvement in language and speech and trying to attain next mile stones. Expressive speech takes time for improvement, vocabulary output is seen only after 3 to 4 months of starting treatment. What else is needed for happiness? But there is also a sense of guilt for losing the valuable time period. There is also a tendency among practicing doctors to attribute everything to the primary diagnosis of CP and not looking for anything else. Always look for additional insult like hypothyroidism creeping up. Vitamin D as a culprit in developmental delay or language delay or in early autism has not being recognised. Let this book bring more light into this. My experience had taught me to look for additional insults occurring (hypothyroidism and vitamin D deficiency) at regular intervals.

Vitamin D should be looked as a "hormone" produced from skin after sunlight exposure due to its multitude of actions on the cells. Due to its nuclear receptor actions every cell in the body needs it for its functioning, due to the recent life style changes vitamin D deficiency has come up as an epidemic in the form of new diseases. **There is a surge in the cases of hypothyroidism recently whether this due to rampant vitamin D deficiency needs investigations**. Other common findings seen is low consistent hemoglobin values with low vitamin D values. Whether these are linked due to low cellular function needs thorough studies. When there is vitamin D deficiency the cells are in a lazy mood and all cellular functions are in slow motion.

Our understanding of mechanism of action and our arbitrary cut off for normal values have limitations. This is a hidden truth. Just go through the steps in the molecular mechanism of action of TSH at nuclear level, we will be astonished by its complexity. Any hormones or chemicals acting through nuclear receptors are complex in nature and have multiple sites for action, that is why it is acting through a common central point in the nucleus. So, all cells will have receptors, and actions will have multiplier effect. Nuclear receptor acting chemicals are, thyroxine, vitamin D, steroid hormones etc. These have varied levels of action in the body. In the case of vitamin D we have not yet recognise its potentials. We can use the recommended cut off for most of the normal cases but when it comes to developmental delay, we have to be more flexible. It will take decades before we arrive at the correct cut off values. Doctors are not in a position to draw definite line for cut offs. Most cut off values are derived taking into consideration 2-SD values or 95 percentiles of values from target population. There are 2.5 percentile of values on either side of bell-shaped nomogram which are not considered. Is it not an arbitrary cut off? We don't know whether these values are actually outside or inside normal range for that particular baby, because each and every individual is different genetically. If you are taking TSH cut off as 4 IU/ml and a child with TSH value 3.8 IU/ml as

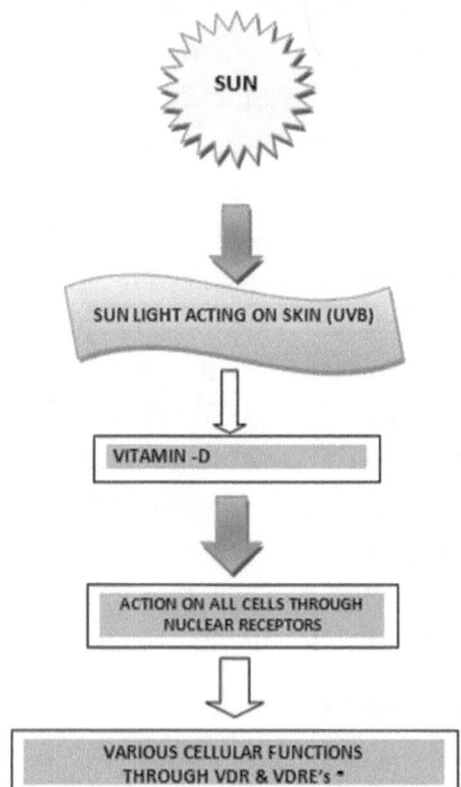

**Figure: 2** Mechanism of action of Vitamin D (*VDR- vitamin D receptors, VDRE's – Vitamin D response elements)

normal, can you guarantee with 100% surety that this value is normal, no, nobody is sure of that. If that baby with TSH of 3.8 IU/ml shows developmental delay, you have to give a trial of thyroxine for you to convince yourself. No RCT in the world is going to do justice for that child. Only way to properly know is to give the benefit of doubt to the compromised baby. Treat for a certain period of time and then see the clinical response and then take a final call.

Technically speaking one molecule is enough to get attached to the receptor for action so, the number of molecules required for all receptors to function is equal to the number of receptors present that is a very small number. (insulin requirement = number of insulin receptors, but that is not true). But that is not the case in practice, it is the concentration of the molecule that is important for any chemical interaction, molecule – receptor interaction to take place (molecular random movement, collision, chance interaction with receptors, half-life of compound all these factors come into play). That is why blood levels of molecules are very important and the efficiency of this interaction is depend on many unknown factors. At which particular concentration the interactions are optimal can vary from individual to individual so drawing a strict line is foolish from our part. Frankly we don't have a full idea of these factors and so our cut offs values have limitations. So, we cannot say with 100% accuracy that a particular cut off value is cent percent correct. This is the reason to suggest when it comes to borderline cases, we have to give the benefit of doubt to the patient to see the response.

**Points regarding thyroxine:**

- In neural cells T3 may control around 5% of all expressed genes and as much as one third of them may be regulated directly at the transcriptional level.

- Mutation in the Monocarboxylate transporter-8 causing a severe retardation of development and neurologic impairment, likely due to deficient T4, T3 transport to the brain.

**Different types of clinical presentation of development delay are discussed below.**

1. Eight months preterm baby (32weeks) coming at 3 months of postnatal age with complaints of lack of social smile. Here chronologic age is 3 months and corrected date of birth (CDOB) is 1 month. It will take one more month to reach the upper age

limit for social smile to attain, so, give one more month to the baby, but make sure to review after one month.

2. Full term baby coming at 2 months of age with no face regard or social smile. it's worrisome and should start investigations to find out the cause.

3. Full term baby coming at 2 months of age with face regard (that means looking at face) but with no social smile. Once face regard comes most babies will smile at you in around 15 to 20 days' time, so ask to follow up after a month.

4. The following conditions are worrisome and should take necessary actions.

    a. No social smile by 2 months corrected age (CDOB)
    b. Not opening hands by 2 months (persistent clinched fist)
    c. Persistent Retrocolis (excessive arching of back) abnormal
    d. No supine to prone by 4 months
    e. No head control by 6 months
    f. No sitting by 9 months
    g. No independent standing by 1 year
    h. No independent walking by 1 year 2 months
    i. No running by 2 years
    j. No pincer grasp by 1-1/4 years
    k. No speech by 1 year
    l. Only 2 words by 1-1/2 years
    m. Paucity of words by 2 years
    n. No joining of 2 words by 2-1/2 years

o. No joining of 3 words by 3-1/2 years

p. Hand preference before 2 years

q. Compared to sibling this child is delayed

r. Compared to the other twin this child is delayed

s. Any regression or loss of milestones

t. Excessive leg tightness any age (difficulty in putting diapers, scissoring)

u. Excessive floppiness at any age.

v. Any autistic tendencies (self-play, not interacting with environment or people, excessive hand regard, repetitive actions, repetitive words, no eye contact, into his own world, lack of speech development etc)

w. Squint persisting after 6 months (squint up to 6 months is normal as binocular vision starts only by 4 months of age)

x. Inconsolable cry, any regularly appearing abnormal movements or changes in tone apart from seizures.

y. Any time seizure is abnormal and needs detailed investigations, except for typical febrile seizures.

z. Any abnormal smell for baby or urine

aa. Prolonged periods of constipation

ab. Any time pale coloured stool, prolonged jaundice persisting beyond one month of age.

ac. Excessive aggressiveness

ad. Any recent behavioural change

5. A 2-year-old child coming from gulf with speech delay and lack of social interactions. This is a clear case of lack of social

interactions from parents. Father will be away for job, mother mostly in kitchen and doing her daily works, no grandparents so child is left unattended or left Infront of TV or mobile. For these children do basic development delay screening, and you can see that invariably vitamin D levels will be very low. Some of these children also shows autistic features as mentioned above and responds well to treatment. Most children respond well to just vitamin D treatment alone. Treatment should be with appropriate dose for prolonged duration. I have seen several children receiving inadequate treatment and seeing no desired results.

6. Child coming to you with an array of investigations for developmental delay at 1-1/2 or 2 years of age. They would have consulted many doctors on the way, what I have noticed is some of the borderline values of TSH were overlooked and sometimes free T4 and vitamin D values are not checked. (doctors have not started correlating development delay and speech delay with vitamin D deficiency). Over looked TSH values are in the range of 4.5, 4.9 etc. for the child these mild deviations can cause havoc on development. One more added insult is not starting intensive physiotherapy (early intervention) for these children. Pathetic to see a child who is still crawling at 1-1/2 years of age and not getting early interventions. Once you start corrective measure these children starts to improve, as a doctor you are satisfied and parents are also happy. Degree of improvement varies. But always there is a regret of lost golden time period. This is the exact reason for writing this book. Never overlook important critical values, need to have lower cut offs for TSH, always do free T4, and vitamin D estimations. Treat vitamin D deficiency with adequate doses for sufficient duration of time. (higher levels needed to attain for good response, from my experience level >60 nmol/L is adequate). There is an exaggerated worry about toxic doses, in my opinion it is not

true. Since vitamin D has its action at nuclear receptors, hundreds and hundreds of genes may be activated and vitamin D may be making fundamental changes in CNS like myelination, synaptic connections, improved functions of neurons.

a. So how to treat the following case: age 1-1/2 years, 8.9 Kg, hypertonia, only sitting with support, no language development, with chest deformity of rickets. The investigation values are: TSH 4.2, T4- 8.4ug/ml, FreeT4 – 0.89ng/ml, vitamin D 13.4 IU/ml, Hb-9.8.

b. This is a clear case of hypothyroidism with vitamin D deficiency with anaemia.

c. Start with Tab: Thyroxine 25 mic once daily early morning empty stomach diluted in boiled and cooled water (tell parents not to give in milk, absorption can be erratic)

d. Vitamin D preparation 800 IU/ml, 2 ml once daily. (there are no definite recommendations in developmental delay cases) (see table-1)

e. Syp Arachitol (60,000 IU/5 ml), 2.5 ml weekly to be continued or Injection vitamin D 6 lakh IM at 2 to 3 monthly intervals. (injections has the fastest response for developmental delay and rickets)

f. Calcium syrup twice or thrice daily to be continued (after starting vitamin D calcium assimilation into the bone increases and calcium requirement increases, so definitely add calcium supplementation).

g. Repeat TSH, Free T4, after 2 months to adjust the dose to keep TSH below 2.5 and to bring Free T4 above 1.2 ng/ml. From experience it is seen that free T4 values below 1.2 ng/ml can show development lag in at least some cases, so any value below 1.2ng/ml should be aggressively managed for a child who is already showing developmental lag. Once TSH value is stabilized do TSH, free T4 once in 4 to 6 months.

h. There is no need to repeat vitamin D as levels if you are giving adequate doses (daily maintenance with weekly or fortnightly boluses with vitamin D 60,000 IU/5 ml)). The levels can be on the higher side and seeing higher values you may be forced to stop vitamin D, more over vitamin D test is expensive. After about 3 to 4 months, you can reduce the dose of syrup Arachitol (60,000 IU/5ml) from weekly doses to fortnightly doses (once in 2 weeks). Please remember and also tell parents that if you stop vitamin D supplementation, levels can again become low in a weeks' time).

i. Encourage sunlight exposure daily.

j. Simultaneously start intensive early intervention programmes.

k. Ask for greater environmental exposure, more social interactions with outside world etc. (take the child to a playschool (Montessori type playschool is preferred) for play and for the development of social interactions).

l. Also start iron supplementation.

m. Once development catch up has achieved try to maintain vitamin D by having daily exposure to sunlight and by providing vitamin D at regular intervals.

n. How long to give thyroxine: very controversial question, what I follow is given below

   i. For our child give thyroxine till the age of 3 years of age and can stop if all milestones are age appropriate. If all age-appropriate milestones are not attained give thyroxine till that is attained.

ii. After stopping thyroxine for 2 months repeat TSH, FreeT4,& T4 and see the values, if the values are borderline or abnormal continue thyroxine for 2 more years. This is because all children are in a growing phase and we don't want to compromise during the growth phase. If thyroxine values are normal and development milestones are age appropriate you can comfortably stop thyroxine but repeat TSH, free T4 once in 6 to 12 months period.

**Vitamin D recommendations.**

**Table: 1** (Royal children's Hospital Melbourne Guidelines)

| Classification | Vitamin D levels (nmol/L) | Vitamin D levels (ng/ml) |
| --- | --- | --- |
| Severe deficiency | <12.5 nmol/L | <5 ng/ml |
| Moderate deficiency | 12.5 to 29 nmol/L | 5 to 11.6 ng/ml |
| Mild deficiency | 30 to 49 nmol/L | 12 to 19.6 ng/ml |
| Sufficient | ≥50 nmol/L | ≥20 ng/ml |
| Elevated | ≥250 nmol/L* | ≥100 ng/ml |
| Toxicity is defined as serum 25-OH-D >250 nmol/L (>100 ng/ml) with hypercalcemia and suppression of parathyroid hormone (PTH), PTH flattening happens at 30 ng/ml or 75 nmol/L range. | | |
| Preferred 25 (OH)D range is 40 to 60ng/ml or 100 to 250 nmol/L (Endocrinology society recommendation) | | |

**Vitamin D Preparations available in India.**

- Drops Vitamin D 400 IU/ml and 800 IU/ ml
- Drops Arachitol 60,000/ 5 ml
- SYP Vitamin D 600 IU/5ml, 1000 IU/ 5 ml and 2000 IU/5 ml
- Sachet vitamin D 60000 IU/ sachet

- Tab Vitamin D 2000 IU
- Soft Gel capsules 60,000 IU/ capsule
- Inj. Vitamin D 3 lakh IU/ 1ml and 6 lakh IU/ 1ml
- Multivitamin drops contain 200 IU/ml

**Take home message:**

- Always be sensitive towards parental concern for development delay
- Don't delay investigations whenever there is a doubt on development.
- Always include TSH, FreeT4, T4, T3, vitamin D, Hb in the developmental delay panel along with other tests. (never miss a case of hypothyroidism or vitamin D as a cause for developmental delay)
- Treat in sufficient dose for sufficient duration of time.
- Early interventions to be started early for children with developmental delay
- Encourage sunlight exposure daily.

## Chapter 23

# IN-UTERO SEPSIS-SHOCK-SEQUENCE (SSS) AND DEVELOPMENT DELAY

All are familiar with perinatal insults and later developmental delay. But if the in-uteri insult occurs earlier (days or weeks) the child can recover (partially) from the insult while inside the uterus (but with residual brain damage) and can be born as vigorous baby without requiring any resuscitation, but only to present later with developmental delay. This type of presentation is not very rare but are mostly missed and is very difficult to establish the cause of developmental delay.

## CASE SCENARIO

A FTND, MSAF baby who cried after stimulation, was kept in NICU for 3 days for mild respiratory distress and tachypnea. Baby did not have any features of HIE, but septic work up was positive. Mother had fever with decreased fetal movements 7 days prior to delivery which was treated conservatively. At the time of delivery one week later there was only MSAF as a significant finding. Baby was treated with IV antibiotics for 7 days and was discharged on day 7 of life. MRI was taken at 2 months of life in view of absent social smile at 2 months of life showed a surprising picture of cystic PVL. Child later on developed features of quadriplegic CP with development delay and microcephaly.

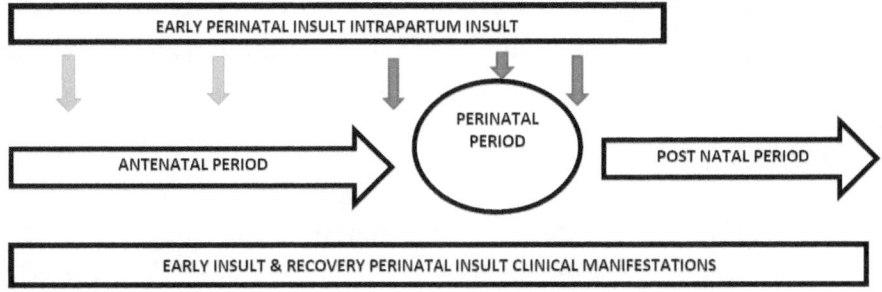

**Figure: 1**   Timing of perinatal insult and recovery.

## DISCUSSION

What happened in the above case is that the baby inside the uteri underwent a perinatal insult earlier, days or weeks before delivery. But due to the time lag in delivering the baby, baby partially recovers from the insult and delivers a near normal baby (doesn't require resuscitation). But actually, carries the scars of pervious insult, manifesting in later life. The external symptoms in mother was fever and fetal distress (decreased fetal movements, tachycardia, bradycardia or passage of meconium). These symptoms in mother was treated conservatively at home or in hospital. Since labor pain was not initiated during that time nobody noticed the event. In the above case child received sufficient insult to produce brain damage, but recovered partially from that insult and by the time child was ready for delivery, child was able to cry with stimulation and no perinatal asphyxia event was documented.

Everybody would have seen this kind of pattern. Several cases of unexplained development delay without any perinatal insult history can be due to these types of early perinatal insults. This can be a case of in-uteri sepsis and damage, but recovers by the time baby was delivered and didn't show any signs of HIE. In uteri damage would have occurred 3 to 5 days or weeks prior to delivery and recovered reasonably well from sepsis. These kinds of antenatal insults can cause intra uterine seizures (equivalent to HIE-2) and recovers by the time baby is ready for delivery.

## INTRODUCTION

In-utero sepsis is a common topic of discussion but "shock in fetus" is not much discussed topic and here I want to bring to the discussion the importance of shock inside the uterus. Sepsis- shock -sequence (SSS) can occur where ever there is infection and so, that can also occur inside uterus. Everybody is aware of the in-utero sepsis but nobody has thought in detail or in depth beyond that it seems. Several of the neurologic sequalae are unexplained by the perinatal events alone (for example, child having no perinatal insult but developing developmental delay with MRI showing cystic PVL). Generally, obstetricians are much concerned about problems related to mother and less concerned about infections in the newborn. They are mainly concerned about the primary symptoms like decreased fetal movements and they are happy if fetus is relieved of that symptoms and won't go beyond that. A fetus producing decreased fetal movement due to infection is not relieved of infection even if the fetal movements return to normal. (Also read the chapters on shock to know the mechanisms of damage occurring during shock).

Fetus inside uterus can get infection like any newborn baby. Baby inside the uterus is in a sterile environment and is protected by several layers of membrane, more over it has the protection of maternal immunity against microorganisms. Infection can come from different directions like ascending infection from cervical canal (through intact membranes) into the amniotic fluid and from there to the GIT and lungs of the fetus, finally into the blood stream. Hematogenous spread from mother can occur whenever there is bacteremia Any fever in mother is accompanied by bacteremia during the early phase. Any chronic infection in the mother even when asymptomatic (chronic dental caries, asymptomatic UTI) is accompanied by bacteremia. Rupture of the membrane increases the chances of infection but studies has shown that organism can pass through intact membranes. What happens when an organism attacks a 37 weeks old fetus?

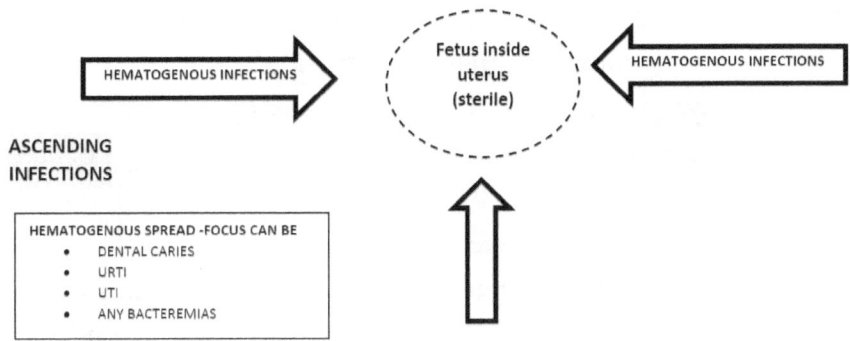

**Figure: 2** Different modes of infection in a fetus.

**Source of infection and maternal and fetal symptoms,**

- Mild maternal fever for few days or cough and cold for 3 to 5 days
- Asymptomatic or symptomatic URTI in mother.
- Dental caries
- Asymptomatic or symptomatic UTI in mother.
- Mother can have LPV, decreased fetal movements, MSAF or oligohydramnios
- Fetus can have tachyarrhythmias, CTG variations etc.
- Investigations can show elevated WBC counts, elevated CRP, UTI, HVS showing growth of pathogenic organisms.
- Abnormal weight gain for fetus (fetal oedema) or IUGR or flattening of weight gain.
- USG showing oligohydramnios from decreased fetal urine output.

How are these symptoms produced? let us discuss the mechanism of each symptoms.

## Sepsis & Shock like situation in the fetus:

Once the organisms breach the protective barrier and reach the fetus, its further course is comparatively easy as fetal immune system is immature. Then organisms multiply and releases endotoxins and fetal immune system produces inflammatory mediators for mobilizing the immune system. These inflammatory mediators and endotoxins produce a shock like condition with capillary leakage, decreased circulating blood volume, low BP, with resultant compromise on organ perfusion. Only opposing factors are circulating maternal antibodies against this particular organism. There can be compensatory tachycardia, counter regulatory hormone release etc. Decreased Kidney blood flow causes decrease in fetal urine output manifested externally as gradual decrease in amniotic fluid volume, later leading on to oligohydramnios. Moreover, there are circulating antibody against all common organisms in fetal blood from maternal circulation which prevents unchecked multiplication of organisms. Whenever fetal circulating volume decreases (early shock) compensatory mechanisms kicks in there by there is tachycardia, renin-angiotensin aldosterone axis activation and kidney start to conserve water and also increases the perfusion pressure to the organs. Like outside, inside uterus there is preferential shunting of blood from non-vital centers (skin, GIT, muscles) to vital centers like brain, heart and kidneys. Babies with long-term oligohydramnios presents with wrinkled skin (with poor subcutaneous fat), poor muscle mass, very low glycogen reserves in the liver etc. So, any drastic variation in amniotic fluid volume or oligohydramnios is a worrisome sign.

If the infection and shock worsen then organ perfusion gets compromised and brain damage can occur. I will explain little bit more. When shock is developing there is shunting of blood from non-vital organs to vital organs and in the vital organs like brain there is internal redistribution of blood from non-vital centers to vital centers. So, blood gets diverted from white matter areas, periventricular areas to brain stem, basal ganglia etc. if this mechanism is prolonged or becomes severe, it causes serious damage to the non-vital areas. They manifest as various degrees of PVL. So, not all PVL are produced after birth some are definitely produced before birth. In these poorly perfused areas, there occurs the phenomenon called "tissue level hypoglycemia" which is discussed in detail in the chapters on shock. There is tissue level hypoglycemia and hypoxemia associated with shock. Here tissue level hypoglycemia and hypoxemia occur even when blood level of glucose are normal. This causes severe cellular damage through ATP deficiency, cell membrane disruption, accumulation of excitatory neurotransmitter (glutamate) etc. If these insults were of short duration then the damages are subtle and reversible. But if the events are prolonged then the damages are severe and permanent. This highlights the importance of active interventions when there are even subtle signs of fetal compromise. When dealing with fetal distress think of the mechanisms of neuro-destructions and adjustments the baby is undergoing and the damage it causes to the fetus. Then we will be forced to take quick actions. Always remember, severity of brain damage from shock is proportional to the degree of shock and duration of shock

> Brain damage due to shock ∞ Duration and severity of shock

So, a mild shock (subtle shock or compensatory shock) for prolonged period produces same damage as severe shock of shorter duration. We always give importance to moderate or severe shock. So compensatory stage of shock is not good for long term as there are area in the brain compromised during compensated shock (periventricular white matter areas and any areas of brain are vulnerable, our ability to measure the damages is highly restricted).

Sepsis manifestations can be skin oedema, sudden increase in weight, sometimes even hydrops, stress causing in-uteri passage of meconium, decreased fetal activity manifested as decreased fetal movements. Some associated additional insults like in-utero hypoglycemia is also a possibility which can aggravate brain damage, more over these are unmeasurable. So, in-uteri shock is a real possibility and we are not giving much importance to its symptoms. These can have long term implications after birth. Fetal scalp VBG can show increasing metabolic acidosis. We have to corelate fetal signs and symptoms with underlying pathophysiology.

Most mothers would have developed antibody against most commensal and common organisms and also against recently exposed organisms, which renders the fetus some protection against the invading organism from circulating antibodies. But if mother gets a new variety of infections (like new hospital acquired pathogens) then organisms can multiply rapidly unchecked causing more problems to the fetus. For clarity purpose I have categorized in-uteri sepsis and shock into different stages depending on its severity (stage -0, 1, 2, 3), stage -0 is mild and stage -3 is the severest. Table-1 shows the different stages of shock, pathophysiology, signs and symptoms, and consequences.

**Table: 1** In-Utero Sepsis Shock, Pathophysiology and Consequences

| Stages of In-Utero Sepsis-Shock Sequence (SSS) | Pathophysiology | Signs and Symptoms (Maternal & Fetal) | Consequences |
|---|---|---|---|
| Asymptomatic infections (Stage-0) | Not much pathological changes in-uteri | Nil or subtle fever, no fetal signs like tachyarrhythmias | After birth baby can present with sepsis, pneumonia, immediately or within few days |
| Early infections (Stage-1) | Mild circulatory deficiencies, stress, release of counter hormones (Renin-Angiotensin-Aldosterone (RAA) axis stimulation) | Fetal tachycardia or bradycardia, decreased fetal urine manifested as oligohydramnios MSAF, CTG variations | Born as sepsis-shock, pneumonia, MAS, with low APGAR score. |
| Moderately advanced fetal infections (In-utero BP maintained) (Stage-2) | Fetal shock causes hypoxia-hypoglycemia* to the brain, resulting in brain damage, fetal seizures, fetal distress and passage of meconium. | Advanced CTG variations, decreased FM, thick MSAF, low APGAR score at birth | Sever sepsis and shock and pneumonia, advanced HIE, seizures, high risk for long term neurodevelopmental consequences even without h/o HIE. |

| Stages of In-Utero Sepsis-Shock Sequence (SSS) | Pathophysiology | Signs and Symptoms (Maternal & Fetal) | Consequences |
|---|---|---|---|
| Severe fetal infection and shock (In-Utero BP fall) (Stage-3) | Fetal bradycardia and arrest, hydrops, in-utero demise | Absent FM, born as severely depressed baby, goes into advanced HIE | Long term neurologic damage, advanced stages of HIE, seizures, severe sepsis |

**Notes:** One of the things happening and not discussed widely is these children can recover from these episodes of sepsis-shock-sequence and child can have normal CTG and is born normally without HIE. This past episode is forgotten and delivered several days or weeks later only to present later with neurodevelopmental delay, microcephaly. This child will never have recorded HIE history. MRI shows gross abnormality of neuronal losses and damage.

- IN-UTERO INFECTIONS →
  - SEPSIS -SHOCK- SEQUENCE (SSS) →
    - ORGAN COMPROMISES →
      - SIGNS AND SYMPTOMS →
        - ADVANCED ORGAN DAMAGE →
          - LONG TERM CONSEQUENCES OR FETAL DEMISE

There is a lack of clinicopathological correlation with the signs and symptoms in mother and fetus with the undergoing pathological process. If you are aware of the pathological process undergoing you will be on more alert and your actions will be prompter and quicker. If you are not thinking about the pathological process behind a decreased fetal movement you will take everything callously. If you are aware that muscles and brain are weak due to hypoxia and more advanced hypoxia can jeopardize everything can prompt you to take action. Similarly, awareness that MSAF is due to extreme stress on fetus will prompt you to take action. This callous nature from the part of healthcare provided is due to the fact that only a very low fraction of calls for fetal distress (↓FM, MSAF, oligohydramnios etc.) ends in serious neonatal problems. Majority of in-uteri abnormalities are solved well properly after birth. Only occasional babies end up requiring significant resuscitation (1 per 1000 deliveries). That is taken as normal occurrence and non-preventable whatever precaution you take. More over obstetric doctors are not aware about the long-term consequences for their babies because of lack of feedback. Even pediatricians are not able to co-relate well with the developmental consequences.

**Table: 2** Clinicopathological Co-relation

| Clinical condition | Underlying pathology | Long term consequences & remedial measures |
|---|---|---|
| **Decreased fetal movements (↓FM)** | Due to multitude of causes child is too weak to move normally, can be due hypoxia, tissue level hypoglycemia from shock, or as part of sepsis and shock. (activity of any child /fetus decreases with infections) | → It is an early sign if it is prolonged or associated with other signs and symptoms can have long term neurological consequences. → closely follow and intervene accordingly |
| **MSAF** | Due to extreme fetal stress, fetus relaxes anal sphincter. (During hanging like events, the victim passes motion and urine, the stress for the fetus may be similar, who knows). Stress can be from infection, shock, hypoxia. In post-date MSAF is a natural phenomenon. | → Two points (1), degree of stress needed for meconium passage and its damage, (2), consequences of meconium aspiration and its problems |
| **Oligohydramnios** <br> →**Chronic** <br> →**Acute** | **Chronic** -due to IUGR, HTN, serious renal anomaly and chronic infections <br><br> **Acute** -is due to sepsis-shock-sequence related decreased urine output. Renin-angiotensin axis activation. | Both can have long term neurodevelopment consequences. In C/C cases there is more time for adaptations to occur, but acute can be more damaging because lack of time for adaptation |

| Clinical condition | Underlying pathology | Long term consequences & remedial measures |
|---|---|---|
| **Scar tenderness** | Is a reasonably good sign of in-uteri infections, and early intervention is warranted. Otherwise more serious complications of uterine rupture and advanced infection can occur. Indicates infection has reached previous scar site. | Long term consequences depend on the complications |
| **CTG variations**<br>→Less serious<br>→variations | **Non-reactive or inadequate NST** / Absent beat to beat variability with fetal activity | Risk for birth asphyxia (3 in 1000 chance of fetal demise within 1 week following non-reactive NST |
| **CTC variations**<br>→Serious variations | **Type II decelerations or Positive CST**<br><br>Doppler flow abnormalities<br><br>*Indicate uteroplacental insufficiency | High risk for birth asphyxia (88 in 1000 risk for still birth following positive CST + non-reactive NST) |
| **Maternal fever**<br>→1st & 2nd trimester<br>→Last trimester | Maternal fever indicates infection mostly viral infections during early period, can have devastating consequences. 1-2nd TM: At this organ forming stage fetus has no significant defense against organisms so (both viral and bacterial) they will freely multiply and destroy most organs.<br><br>3rd TM: infection produces less organ damage, but can be born with infection | 1-2 trimester infections can have serious consequences, bacterial and viral infections both can cause abortions and those who survive will have serious consequences |

| Clinical condition | Underlying pathology | Long term consequences & remedial measures |
|---|---|---|
| **Maternal UTI**<br>→**Asymptomatic**<br>→**Symptomatic** | Most pregnancy will have asymptomatic infections and are treated conservatively. But sometimes organisms can invade the fetus either through hematogenous or ascending route. Symptomatic infections have more chance of infecting the fetus. But asymptomatic infections have more chance of missing the detection by doctor so increased incidence of in-uteri infection for the fetus. | Both types have the same consequences of in-uteri infection and shock. |
| **Maternal HTN** | Produces restricted nutrient and oxygen availability to the fetus and so there is varying degrees of growth restriction. More chance of producing IUGR babies. | All the consequences of IUGR babies. |
| **IUGR**<br>→**Intrinsic**<br>→**Extrinsic** | **Intrinsic**: genetic defects restrict growth<br><br>**Extrinsic**: outside causes restricting fetal growth, several examples in standard texts. | In intrinsic IUGR growth potential is limited due to genetic defects. Extrinsic growth restriction improves once restrictions for growth are removed. |

| Clinical condition | Underlying pathology | Long term consequences & remedial measures |
|---|---|---|
| **Non progress of labor unrelated to CPD** | Activation of fetal Hypothalamic - Pituitary- Adrenal axis activation is necessary for the normal labor progression. (in the absence of CPD). infection may have a role in this. | Depends on the degree of infection to the fetus |
| **A/c insult Vs c/c insult**<br><br>a/c fetal insults like cord prolapse, placental abruption, tightening cord around the neck & cord knot | **A/c insults:** like cord prolapse there is no time for the **diving reflex** to occur in the brain. (*diving reflex: where by vital areas of the brain (brain stem) gets blood supply by diverting blood from less vital areas, like cerebral cortex*). So vital area suffers more.<br><br>C/C insult: hypertension, intermittent cord compression | In a/c insults brain stem suffers more so presents with apnea in the immediate newborn period.<br><br>But in c/c insults like slow cord compression, diving reflex occurs and vital areas are spared and cerebral cortex suffers more and presents with seizures. |

This chapter is written to make more people aware of the in-utero consequences of shock. Please remember that **Shock and hypoglycemia can also occur inside the uterus**. Like outside sepsis associated hypoglycemia, inside uterus also sepsis associated hypoglycemia can occur, who is going to correct this, nobody will notice this silent damage and all can end up as idiopathic developmental delay. Shock associated tissue level hypoglycemia can also occur inside uterus. In-utero sepsis is a problem but most of us won't think deep into its pathogenesis and consequences. If you are aware of the consequences, we will become more vigilant and we will be forced to take actions early. Our curiosity should take us to dig deep inside each of the symptoms the fetus produces. Once you realize the deep underlying pathophysiology you will be forced to act responsibly. Decreased fetal movements, decreased urine out, heart rate variations, meconium passage all are distress calls from the fetus, take utmost care in handling these calls. Don't be a part in making more CP babies but rather partner in reducing incidence of CP.

# Chapter 24

# IS ECZEMA ALWAYS AN "ALLERGIC" CHRONIC DISEASE OR A TREATABLE DISEASE?

This chapter discusses my different view on eczema. There is a tendency now a days to label every skin lesion which are chronic to label as eczema. We all know skin lesions won't get cured by its own without proper treatment. First the diagnosis should be correct. Lots of fungal lesions are misdiagnosed and labelled as eczema and treated with highly potent steroids and emollients for long duration without a permanent cure. Any lesions will show decrease in inflammations and itching once steroids are applied, that doesn't mean it is cured and recur once steroids are stopped. Have seen few children coming to us with cushingoid features after prolonged topic application of steroid (Betamethasone valerate) for almost a year!

Different kinds of skin infections show different predilection during a year, with pyoderma occurring more towards summer months and fungal infections during dry winter months. My hypothesis for this increased fungal infection during winter season is the following. Due to constant exposure to dry, cold wind, skin becomes dry and starts to produce microscopic cracks. Into these breaks atmospheric fungal spores gets deposited and they grow and multiply there. Once infection settles immune mobilization and inflammation kick starts and redness, itching, lichenification and scaling develops. Itching produces deeper cracks and organism settles into more deeper tissues. Dermatophytes penetrates deep inside the skin, skin hardens, oozing and crusting seen, degree of itching and the degree of immune reaction elicited by the body all depends on the nature of organism. This skin dermatophyte infection is first seen (mother lesion) usually over the shin and cheek areas. These are the maximum wind exposed areas and are more prone for dryness. From these mother lesions fungal infections spreads to surrounding areas. But candida infection first appears in the wet flexural creases like neck, cubital fossa, inguinal areas, they need moisture for growth. You can clearly see this pattern if you ask a detailed history. If you apply steroids at this stage inflammation subsides and patients feel better, but only to recur after stopping steroids because dermatophytes remain in the skin unaffected. Steroid wipes out all the inflammatory reactions and skin appears smoother and patients feels better. These kinds of skin lesion should not be labeled as allergic to breast milk (rash on cheek of breastfeeding babies) or allergy to cow's milk etc. before ruling out primary fungal infections. Fungal skin infections are more common than absolute allergy to breast milk or cow's milk. When crusting and oozing increases secondary bacterial infections can also settles and the gross picture changes. The organism most commonly encountered are staphylococcus aureus and staphylococcus epidermidis. For superadded secondary bacterial infections give a course of oral ampicillin + cloxacillin combination along with a topical antibacterial cream.

Candida is a common skin pathogen seen during and after newborn period. This usually starts in the flexural areas (presents as red rash with fine nodules in the neck, cubital fossa and inguinal areas) and then spreads to other areas. When spread to wider areas topical treatment becomes difficult. When the involved area becomes very wider, we have to give systemic antifungal agents for 3 to 4 weeks. As the candid skin infection establishes, the skin texture changes, skin's softness disappears, it becomes harder, rougher and drier. Usually, we imply this to the soap we use, soaps also have a role to play in the skin texture production. As the candida infection increases itching, redness appears and scaling increases. As infants cannot itch, they show irritability and fussiness. Usually seen modality of treatment is application of emollients with change to "pharmaceutical" soaps with "pH -o-meter"! Definitely there will be relief to the baby but you cannot stop the emollient application. No problem with this kind of treatment, provided you identify the primary cause and treat that also. Most doctors and even dermatologist (several prescriptions seen) doesn't bother to treat the underlying candid infections (or they are not recognizing the underlying fungal component?). These children carry these lesions for months or for years and skin changes from bad to worse. New diagnostic labels like, eczema, allergic dermatitis, cow's milk allergy, allergy to breast milk etc. appears. The underlying pathology is buried deep inside. I have treated several of these with multiple combinations of oral antifungal agents (fluconazole, Griseofulvin), keratolytic agents (Whitefield ointment), topical antifungal creams (clotrimazole, ketoconazole, terbinafine) emollients and short course of mild steroids (eg. mometasone, to calm down the inflammation and itching). Treated successfully several of these very long duration (3 to 11 years) cases of skin lesions labelled as "eczema" with topical application and systemic antifungals for complete cure. Supplementing these treatments with vitamin D preparations fastens healing. Rarely we get non-infectious eczema cases, buts its numbers are really small. My point is most so-called eczema cases responds well once you treat the underlying fungal infections. Superficial fungal infection (with no signs of inflammation- redness or itching, e.g. Tinea versicolor, T. alba) only need topical antifungal or topical keratolytic agents. Deep fungal infections with local inflammations and nail fungal infections need oral antifungal medications along with topical agents.

Antifungal treatment should be of sufficiently long duration till complete cure is attained. Otherwise, lesions reappear once you stop treatment. Duration of treatment can vary from one month to a year. Toe nail infection need treatment up to a year. Do regular follow up and continue treatment till all traces of infections are removed. One more practical point to emphasis is, I usually change the soap used to another brand to change the texture (nature) of the skin. Different soaps have different fat moiety and pH content. This strategy is very useful in rapidly spreading candid infection of the skin, multiple site Tinea versicolor or T. alba infections. The rapid spreading of the above-mentioned infection is due to the favorable nature of the skin for these organisms, so by changing soap to another brand the skin texture changes and that make life difficult for the fungus to grow and they cannot flourish any longer. This strategy is useless for deeply rooted infections (fig-1).

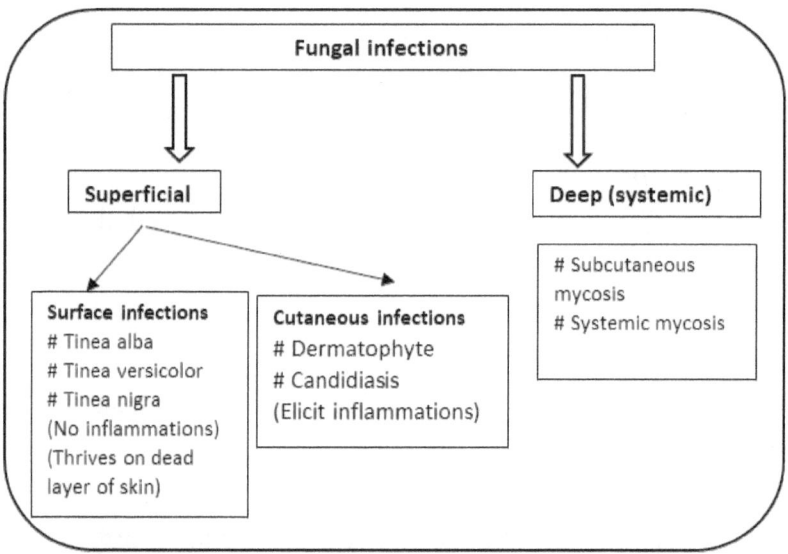

**Figure -1**   Fungal Infections of skin (Mycosis)

**Table: 1** Types of Skin Infections and Treatment Strategies.

| Type of skin infections | Features | Treatment |
|---|---|---|
| Superficial fungal infections eg. Tinea alba and T. Versicolor | Since the infection is superficial (in the superficial dead epithelium) there are no associated inflammatory reactions | Apply antifungal cream or white field ointment for 3 to 6 weeks (white field ointment is the best) Vitamin D is very helpful Change your skin texture by changing to a new soap brand*. |
| Deeper skin infection: Dermatophyte, tinea infections (T. corporis, T.pedis etc.), candidiasis | Signs of inflammation present: itching, redness, scaling etc. (Sometimes very extensive and deep dermatophyte infections doesn't respond well to topical antifungal cream, here we have to use systemic antifungal and mild topical steroid ointments) | Antifungal ±white field ointment for sufficient duration (4 to 16 weeks) Antibacterial cream for superadded infections Emollients for reducing dryness, scaling and itching Short duration mild topical steroids like mometasone cream to decrease the inflammations Vitamin D supplementation can help in healing Oral fluconazole or Griseofulvin for severe extensive & deep cases |

\* Logic is, the fungus which was growing comfortably cannot grow on an altered environment of the skin by changing its texture by changing over to a new brand of soap. Soaps can give varying skin textures by its difference fat moiety and pH content.

My point in writing this chapter is, before labeling any skin lesion as eczema due to allergy please try to rule out any fungal infections as the triggering factor. Most of the time it used to be a fungal infection.

Ask specifically for its evolution and nature of spread. Young children's cheek is a favorite site and before labelling it as milk allergy try with antifungal and emollient creams for sufficient duration of time. (Chronic subclinical bacterial throat infection can also produce cheek rash in babies, as the infected saliva constantly irritate the skin). The duration of treatment depends on the skin turnover time for a cell to reach from basal layer of dermis to the superficial layer till it is shredded out. Face has the fastest turnaround time of less than a month and palms and soles may take many months, finger nails and toe nails takes 6 months to 1 year. Your treatment duration also has to extend that much of time.

Recently seen a 5 month of child on treatment for "eczema" with oral prednisolone for 2 months from a reputed skin specialist. Worried parents approached me when the specialist doctor told to continue prednisolone for one more month. Is this treatment strategy justified without treating the underlying primary cause and using systemic steroids for such a long time for an infant? From history it was only a candid rash spread from neck and inguinal area and spreaded extensively. Any inflammation under the sun subsides with steroids but only to recur later on stopping it.

Anything identified as foreign by the body will trigger an immune attack to contain or destroy it. That can be bacteria, fungus, protozoa, non-living things like metals (nickel), compounds like penicillin, chemicals in food items, preservatives, coloring agents etc. the list is endless. Our aim is to find the primary trigger and remove it. Pointers to trigger we can get from history, nature of spread, similar history in other family members etc. Justified in giving a short course of steroid if symptoms are severe. So, before labelling any skin lesion as a dead entity like eczema try to find the root cause and treat that for a permanent cure.

## Chapter 25

# HOW TO HANDLE THE COMPLAIN OF LOSS OF APPETITE IN A CHILD?

Loss of appetite is a common complaint by parents and is true most of the time. With proper history and examination, we can find out the cause and advise remedial measures. Most of the children thrives well on breastfeeding till 6 months of age, and mostly the growth faltering happens after 6 months when weaning foods are introduced. Is it late to start weaning food at 6 months? This is a controversial question and need debates, I personally want to start weaning by 4 to 4-1/2 months as weaning takes time, mother and baby needs to adapt. Most mothers are not smart enough to start proper weaning instantaneously. If you start weaning by 6 months and everything goes well it takes at least 2 months to establish proper weaning. Most of the time there is growth faltering happening, that is the reason for me to bring up this controversial topic. Through debates between experts new normal can be reached. Following are the problems child and parents' encounter during weaning.

1. Most mothers don't know how to prepare proper weaning foods. This is a collateral damage of loss of joint family system.
2. Child becomes too much demanding by 4 to 5 months of age and parents may be forced to opt for top feeds (mostly with a bottle) as it is forbidden to give early weaning foods.
3. Giving too much diluted feeds
4. Giving too much water in between feeds especially with a bottle leads to growth flattening.

5. Don't know how to prepare healthy weaning foods without contamination.
6. Don't know the concept of slowly increasing consistency of weaning food from liquid to semi solid to solid foods, from mono cereals to cereal-pulse combination to multi cereals.
7. Things happening after introduction of improper weaning foods and techniques.
    a. Growth flattening
    b. Increased episodes of infections, both diarrhea and upper respiratory tract infections from improperly prepared food.
    c. Loss of appetite following clinical or subclinical infections.
    d. Complaints like, nausea, vomiting, abdominal discomfort, abdominal distension, constipation etc.
8. Increased hospitalizations due to various causes (infections, incessant cry, growth failure)
9. Cultural practices delaying weaning, like rice giving ceremony postponing to 1 year of age due to some inconvenience.

It is a known fact that during the first 6 months of breastfeeding the growth of the child is excellent, the problem comes when weaning is started. During weaning several factors come into play. If one can start weaning a month earlier the people involved can get some training, child also used to know the taste. If properly instructed we can avoid growth flattering after 6 months. A visit to pediatrician around 6 months of age can rectify most of the weaning related problems. Usually after 14 weeks vaccination baby is seen by doctors only around 9 months of age for MMR vaccination. By that time either weaning is established very well or weight gain has flattened from improper weaning. To bring back a flattened growth curve back to normal path is a mammoth task. So, is it time to consider weaning a bit earlier to prevent growth flattening? It is a highly controversial topic, since this book is full of controversial topics one more topic won't cause much of a problem.

Coming to the main topic of loss of appetite in a child, this is a ubiquitous problem with numerous causes. The common reasons are,

1. Improper weaning methods and food preparations
2. Milk addictions and so not taking other foods
3. Excessive liquid-based diets, giving excessive water in between feeds with a feeding bottle, excessively smashed diets
4. Excessive night time breast feeding so not taking food during day time (GIT needs rest it cannot work 24 x7, so, appetite for food decreases during daytime, a commonly observable thing)
5. Recurrent infections especially upper respiratory tract infections lead to low appetite.
6. Asymptomatic URTI can cause low appetite
7. Giving too much diluted feeds
8. Giving excessive water very frequently
9. Hypothyroidism
10. Other undetected chronic infections anywhere (eg. primary complex)
11. Chronic vomiting, constipations etc. (these can be manifestations of chronic infections)

It is obvious from the above list of causes that there is a group of asymptomatic upper respiratory tract infections causing loss of appetite in a child. Asymptomatic is a relative term, some symptoms are there if you ask in detail. The symptoms of infection are mostly overlooked when a parent come with loss of appetite in a child. These subtle infections continuously produce mucoid secretions which are swallowed into the stomach and produce continuous bloating of the abdomen, may have occasional nausea and vomiting. This nausea and vomiting are more in the morning due to the overnight accumulated secretions in the stomach. Continuous stream of organisms also enters the stomach through these secretions. These vomiting episodes are considered as GERD by most doctors and treated accordingly. For me there is no diagnosis of GERD and I rarely give treatment with lansoprazole. For me vomiting is due to some other primary causes like infections, treat that and the vomiting goes away. By this approach there are no chronic vomiting cases for my babies on follow up. My primary approach of treatment is to treat the primary cause and get cured before it becomes chronic.

Immune system is in constant fight with this chronic throat infection even if it is a low profile one. Organisms are also continuously shed into the blood stream, sometimes mother complaints of intermittent feverish nature for her child, these may be periods of bacteremia. Whereever there is infection, however subtle it maybe, child experience loss of appetite and growth failure. It is a known fact that inflammation anywhere in the body causes growth failure and even loss of weight. So, whenever a child comes to you for loss of appetite make a habit to look into the throat using a tongue depressor and enquire about the signs and symptoms of subtle infections. You can see congested enlarged tonsillo-pharyngeal tissue.

**What are the subtle signs and symptoms of "asymptomatic" upper respiratory tract infection?**

- Night time nasal block and disturbed sleep.
- Occasional cough
- Nausea and vomiting especially in the morning
- Foul smelling mouth
- Chronically distended abdomen
- Intermittent abdominal colic and complains of recurrent "gas problem"
- Irregular bowel habits, loose motion or constipation
- Mucoid stools, greenish stools or sometimes blood-stained stools
- Excessive drooling from mouth
- Intermittent fever and cough episodes (exacerbations)
- Slightest provocation produces cough and cold (travel, ice cream, citrus fruits, oil bath, ingestion of grapes, watermelon etc.)
- Intermittent wheezing episodes
- Mostly these patients are labelled "allergic" (chronically inflamed mucosa are hypersensitive to any stimuli, excessive sneezing and nasal discharge are some of its symptoms).
- Loss of appetite, fussy and irritable child (something is constantly irritating the child)

Any of the above complaints should prompt you to look into the throat. If these are infections, take a throat swab for C&S and treat that infections completely and give advice to prevent recurrence. At the same time rule out other causes of loss of appetite. Appetite usually reappears when the infection gets controlled. If the child's weight and height are less than standard, rule out hypothyroidism and vitamin D deficiency.

**TAKE HOME MESSAGE.**

Whenever a child comes with prolonged loss of appetite make a habit of doing throat examination to rule out asymptomatic upper tract infection.

# Chapter 26

# CONSTIPATION: IS SYMPTOMATIC TREATMENT ENOUGH, A DOCTOR'S DILEMMA

Constipation is broadly defined as unsatisfactory defecation characterized by infrequent stools, difficult stool passage or both. Constipation is a common problem encountered throughout life; very serious diseases can present as constipation. In pediatrics, doctors are always in a dilemma to treat or not to treat and how to treat. Only known associations of constipation are formula feeding and hypothyroidism. Different food habits can cause constipation but which food causes definite constipation is not known so a definite association cannot be made. Opposite of constipation is loose motion and which when occurs, treatment is taken promptly because of its messy nature. Always an infection is attributed to it origin. Why can't an infection be a culprit in constipation also? Yes, it can be, this is the topic of discussion of this chapter. My intension is not to list all the known causes of constipation, that you can find in standard text books.

A usual presentation in the OPD is child has not passed stool for the last 3-4 days following an episode of cold and cough. We treat the cold and cough and sometimes the bowel habit returns back to the normal. Some mothers say that after that URI bowel habits are not regular. This observation led me to examine the throat whenever a baby comes with a long history of constipation. Bowel habit definitely changes with URT infection or GIT infection, portal of entry is common for URTI and GIT infections. These infections can end in diarrhea or constipation. Diarrhea will always end up in prompt treatment because of its messy nature and also because of its public awareness abouts its dangers. Constipation on the other hand ends up in mismanagement. The awareness to correlate it with infection is poor among doctors. The following are the different types of manifestations of constipation.

1. Constipation of recent onset of 3-5 days following an upper respiratory tract infection.
2. Constipation of recent onset following introduction of new weaning foods.
3. Intermittent constipation of 3 to 5 months duration without any symptoms.
4. Constipation of 3 to 6 months duration associated with mild intermittent cough and cold and morning nausea and sometimes vomiting.
5. Constipation associated with very poor food intake.
6. Constipation with abdominal distension and thin passage of stools and intermittent leaky button.
7. Very long duration constipation, undernutrition and painful defecation.
8. Child with constipation, developmental lag and ± umbilical hernia
9. Very long duration (1-2 years) of constipation without any symptoms.

Any classic textbook can give you the list of investigations for constipation. Constipation is a fairly common presentation in our OPD. Most doctors treat symptomatically with laxatives and other supportive measures and majority improves with that. My discussion is longstanding constipation which doesn't respond from laxative or other measures. Some type responds well to laxatives only to recur later on stopping laxatives.

Every change in the body has a reason and it is our duty to find the reason and treat accordingly. When your child's complaint is recurrent and long standing never treat only symptomatically, try to find the cause and then treat. Always think out of the box, observing and connecting small thing gives us clues. From my experience constipation is never idiopathic and there are some causes hidden from our view and it is our duty to find it. My observation of altered bowel habits (constipation & diarrhea) with any upper respiratory tract infection led me to think constipation also have an infectious background. I tried to explore the hidden site and most common site turns out to be throat and most had a hidden or sometimes symptomatic infections. My habit of doing throat examinations with tongue depressor in every case of URI help me to cling the association. Most long-term or short-term constipations are associated with upper respiratory tract infections mostly asymptomatic. Symptomatic URTI would have been treated. This observation led to almost > 95% success in finding a permanent cure for constipation. One baseline thing is always rule out hypothyroidism and vitamin-D deficiency along with this. (you may ask why vitamin-D, it is a wonderful "hormone" with versatile actions which I will be discussing in chapters on vitamin-D)

Constipation is change of bowel habit of reduced frequency or passage of hard formed stools with difficulty. Any simple upper respiratory infection can alter your bowel habits and if you don't treat the infection properly it can remain chronic. Organism with its multitude of weapons can do anything. The modern trend in therapeutics is to treat only the symptoms and never to tackle the root causes which caused everything. Usually URTI presents with fever, cough, nasal block, nasal discharges and vomiting and most of these symptoms subside in a week time without much treatment. This is deceptive as there may not be full recovery from infection unless you examine the throat manually. Most throat remains congested with enlarged tonsils; organisms remain there only to be reactivated later upon exposure to cold or for that matter any trigger. Parents may forget this episode of infection and these children may later presents with constipation. If you examine the throat you can see the residual infection. These silent infections constantly seed the gut with organisms and also stimulate mucosal layer to secrete mucoid secretions. These secretions along with chemicals produced by organisms may be affecting the Meissner's and myenteric plexus (or Auerbach's plexus) of the gut to produce immobility.

Majority of doctors will be reluctant to treat this. I treated these completely and found encouraging results. Treatment should not end with ampicillin or azithromycin. You will not find any response with these antibiotics as you are dealing with chronic infections. Most of the time you have to upgrade your antibiotics. Do throat swab for culture and sensitivity in the beginning and it may help you in treatment. You may find resistant organisms or mixed type of growths. The possible organisms are many and few possible organisms and combinations are given below.

- GPC, Penicillin sensitive Streptococci (very rare now)
- GPC, Cloxacillin Sensitive Staph aureus (still very common)
- GPC, Penicillin resistant streptococci or staph aureus (MRSA)
- GPC, penicillin and cephalosporin resistant streptococci or staph aureus
- GPC, MRSA or MRSE
- GNB, E-Coli or Klebsiella resistant to cephalosporin
- GNB, E-Coli or klebsiella highly resistant, only sensitive to fluroquinolones & meropenem
- GPC, GNB, mixed infection with MRSA & MDR Klebsiella
- GPC, GNB MRSA & PDR Pseudomonas

- GNB, PDR pseudomonas sensitive only to polymyxin-B

We do throat swab culture for most throat infections and found out a variety of organism in the cultures. GPC can be streptococci, staph aureus, CONS and sometimes pneumococci. GNB can be E-Coli, Klebsiella, Acinetobacter, Pseudomonas. You have to step up the antibiotics till you attain the cure.

## Let us rewind the normal physiology.

Gastrointestinal tract is wired throughout by sympathetic and parasympathetic nerve fibers and main nerve supply is through Vagus (Parasympathetic). At the local nerve ending there are Meissner's and myenteric plexus (or called Auerbach's plexus).

- **Myenteric plexus or Auerbach's plexus** provides motor innervation to both layers of the muscular layer of the gut, having both parasympathetic and sympathetic fibers (ganglion cell bodies which are present belong to parasympathetic innervation, fibers from sympathetic also reach the plexus). Whereas the submucous plexus (Meissner's plexus) has only parasympathetic fibers and provides secretomotor innervation to the mucosa nearest the lumen of the gut. It arises from cells in the vagal trigone, also known as the nucleus ala cinerea, the parasympathetic nucleus of origin for the tenth cranial nerve, located in the medulla oblongata. The myenteric plexus is the major nerve supply to GIT and controls GI tract motility. According to studies, 30% of the myenteric plexus neurons are enteric secretory neurons thus Auerbach's plexus also has a secretory component. This enteric nervous system (ENS) is known as the "brain of the gut". In Parkinson's disease there is severe constipation.

- **Meissner's plexus or submucous plexus:** this lies in the submucosa of the intestinal wall. The nerves in the plexus are derived from the myenteric plexus which itself is derived from the parasympathetic nerves around the superior mesentery. They contain Dogiel cells and its function is to innervate cells in the epithelial layer and the smooth muscle of the muscularis mucosae. 14% of submucosal plexus neurons are sensory neurons- Dogiel type II, also known as enteric primary afferent neurons or intrinsic primary afferent neurons.

## NORMAL CYCLE OF CONSTIPATION

When a child experience constipation, usually stool hardens and pain is experienced during defecation. Child relates this pain to defecation and child avoids passing motions and he hold backs the stools. This results in harder stools and sometimes this hard stool breaks the mucosa and bleeding occurs during defecation. For any lesions to heal it takes at least a weeks' time, and by that time it is time for next passage of motion this results in further fissuring in the already inflamed area, so pain becomes excruciating. Child completely avoids defecation by not squatting properly, only stands and wiggles. This cycle goes and goes and child also starts to associate passage of motion with food intake and so appetite also decreases. While treating this child we have to break this cycle and reverse all the processes. Points to remember while treating constipation.

1. Emollient or oil application in and around anus for lubrication, this can decrease pain
2. Apply antibacterial + anti-inflammatory ointment in and around the anus till the mucosal lesion heals. (candid-B cream)
3. Stool looseners for sufficient duration (10 to 14 days) and sufficient dose (child should have 1-2 loose stools per day) till the child forgets about the pain. (eg: Smuth, PEG, lactulose)

4. Detect the primary cause and treat (infection, faulty foods, hypothyroidism etc.). mostly it is undetected asymptomatic URTI

5. Daily toilet training around a fixed time so that natural reflexes come normally.

6. Rule out more serious causes like Hirschsprung's disease and other intestinal pathologies.

With this strategy one can treat >90% of cases of constipation seen in OPD permanently, rather than treating constipation symptomatically for months.

**Chapter 27**

# HOW TO LINK GROWTH FAILURE WITH CHRONIC ASYMPTOMATIC AND SYMPTOMATIC THROAT INFECTIONS?

There are several causes for growth failure in a child, before going into more serious causes of growth failure there are very common but undetected causes for growth failure in a child. I will list all the possible causes and discuss in detail the common yet missed varieties which I have observed over the years. I am not in a position to prove these through studies, so, those who sees merit in these can take up and do the studies. Most important one among these is untreated asymptomatic and symptomatic upper respiratory infections. I will also discuss other simple treatable causes of growth failure. Growth failure simply means child is not growing up to his or her potential. There are several charts and tables available for detecting growth failure.

**Common treatable causes of growth failure**

- Hypothyroidism including borderline variety
- Vitamin D deficiency
- Chronic upper respiratory tract infections (asymptomatic and symptomatic)
- Undernutrition
- Growth hormone deficiency
- In-utero infections (TORCH)
- Born as idiopathic IUGR babies

- Genetic syndromes
- Genetic short statures etc.

We will discuss in detail chronic upper respiratory tract infections. Infections in children are common in childhood, mostly they are promptly treated and cured. But sometimes infection becomes chronic, subclinical or symptomatic. Symptomatic infections are usually treated promptly but if the organisms are resistant, they are not completely cured and are most likely to get the label of "allergic". Subclinical infections produce intermittent exacerbations on exposure to cold, ice cream, citrus foods, on travel, or after an oil bath etc. Outcome of URTI can be any of the following,

- Undergoes complete cure
- Becomes a chronic infection with symptoms
- Becomes asymptomatic carrier of infection

If an infection is not treated properly, it gets converted into a chronic infection.

## What are the factors for chronicity?

1. When the organism is resistant to the antibiotics used
2. Incomplete course or under dosing of antibiotics
3. When multiple organisms are present, natural selection occurs
4. When recurrent reinfection is the cause for chronicity then it behaves like chronic infections
5. When infections are labelled as "allergy" then there is no chance for proper cure.
6. When you get highly resistant organisms like MRSA, MDR gram negative organisms, pseudomonas infections the chance for chronicity increases.

7. When you are not doing throat swab culture and sensitivity and you are treating blindly
8. If you don't have the habit of looking the throat with a tongue depressor you never know if the infection has cured or not. Don't always go by symptoms alone.
9. Always try to identify source of infection otherwise destined for recurrence.

**What are the common source of recurrent infections?**

1. Chronically infected family member, carrier family member.
2. Contaminated food items
3. Contaminated water (septic tank near well water)
4. Consuming infection prone food items like grapes, watermelon (due to its large size half of watermelon goes into fridge kept fully expose and the next day comes out as infected).
5. Bad habits like Pica, always putting finger into mouth, mothing of objects.

**Mechanism of growth failure in a child with chronic asymptomatic or symptomatic URTI**

The word asymptomatic infection is relative and if you go into the details, you get subtle signs and symptoms. Once an infection is not cured properly, it establishes inside the lymphoid tissue in the oropharynx, it is not staying there innocently as you think. It is constantly in fight with our immune system. Organisms constantly tries to invade the tissues and blood stream; body continuously fights for its containment. Continuously our system is bombarded with endotoxins, antigens and body continuously produces antibiotics and cytokines against these. It is in dynamic equilibrium and any tilt can produce exacerbation of this already existing infection. The triggering factor can be any cold exposure from ice cream, excess citrus fruits, any superadded viral infections exposing mucosal barriers, any trauma, stress, any intake of infected substances etc. All these actions can give an entry to organism. This is how exacerbations happen.

Let us see how growth failure is produced. As we have discussed subclinical infection is not totally innocent, it is a dynamic equilibrium of fight between organism and body, lots of immune complexes and endotoxins are coming into the blood stream. All these can suppress growth as that occurring in any symptomatic infection. For example, in asymptomatic tuberculosis first manifestation may be growth failure, weight loss and loss of appetite. Same thing is happening in chronic subclinical throat infection. Other mechanisms are, these throat infections constantly produce mucoid secretions in small quantities. These get swallowed into the stomach and produce minor symptoms like nausea, sometimes even vomiting especially in the morning. The morning time vomiting is due to the accumulated secretions from overnight, it wants to get out of the body. Mucinous secretions are indigestible and is converted by colonic bacteria into gas and byproducts. Whenever there is excess mucoid secretions, child feels uncomfortable and will feel gaseous distention, colic abdominal pain. Child gets relief after vomiting, here appetite is severely decreased. Child after taking initial amount of food feels uncomfortable and refuses to take further food, this is the usual complain. There can be exaggerated gastrocolic reflex, which causes abdominal colic from bowel peristalsis.

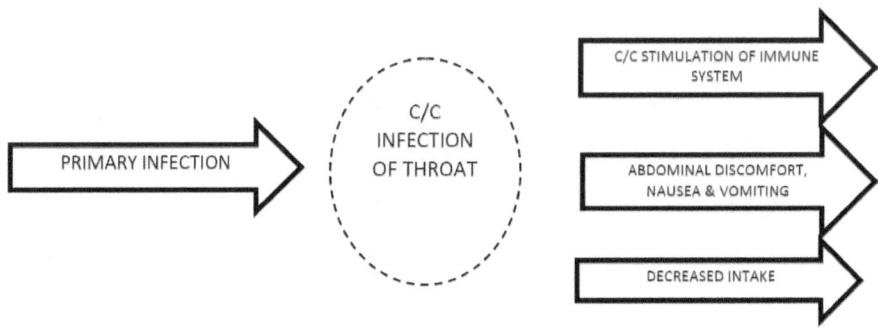

**Figure: 1** Chronic Infection of throat and its actions.

Due to chronic bombardment of organisms from throat, intestine is also under stress, the intestine is also constantly fighting a continuous battle. There can be mesenteric lymphoid hypertrophy due to this chronic infection, which is the usual finding seen in ultrasonography (done for chronic abdominal pain). Child also associates abdominal discomfort with intake of food, so he refuses to take it. He prefers more liquid diet because of less discomfort associated with it, turns to excessive milk addiction, mother is happy to provide more milk as he is not taking any other food.

All the above-mentioned mechanisms result in chronic caloric deficiency and growth failure. There is also excessive metabolic demand happening to fight off the infection. All the mechanisms of weight loss are also happening in chronic subclinical infections but in a reduced scale over a prolonged period, so the net effects are the same.

**How to overcome this trap?**

First of all, you have to convince yourself that there is a trap if primary infection is not cured. Points to avoid this trap and to regain growth momentum.

1. Make a habit of doing throat examinations with a tongue depressor
2. Aim for complete cure of any infections, not just cure of major complaints.
3. While reviewing the case do repeated throat examinations with a tongue depressor for making sure infection has completely cured
4. Don't be in the impression that amoxicillin or azithromycin can cure all the infection in the world. Bacteria are smarter than you think.

5. For infection which are resistant to cure take a throat swab for C&S for better knowing your enemy

6. Try to find out the source of infection, any carriers in the family etc.

7. Treat infections completely.

8. Advise life style modifications, avoiding certain type of foods, avoiding oil applications (oil is a source of infection as organism can freely grow in coconut oil).

9. Advise dietary modifications to increase the caloric intake, in growth failure it is always caloric deficit rather than protein deficiency.

10. Rule out other common causes of growth failure.

11. Maintain a growth chart to know the trajectory.

12. If needed give vitamin supplementations especially vitamin D.

**TAKE HOME MESSAGE**

Any chronic infections in the body can produce growth failure. So, if there is any growth failure in your child ask for any symptoms of chronic URTI and look inside throat with a tongue depressor for detecting any asymptomatic URTI. Most of the time you can find a cause and if you treat that properly, you can see the results. Treatment of these infection can bring back appetite and weight improvement.

## Chapter 28

# INSIGHT INTO COLONIZATION, REINFECTION AND INCOMPLETELY TREATED PRIMARY INFECTION IN A CHILD

Infections in a child is a menacing problem for parents and doctors equally. There are several causes for this increased infection in a child. This can be due to immature immune system, infection prone child's immediate environment, unhygienic foods they consume, child's play and behavioral activities (mouthing), parental insensitiveness towards infections, doctor's treatment approaches etc. Understanding the causes, types of infection, aggressiveness of organisms all are important in its management. Infections has multitude of manifestations in a growing child. A newborn baby can never maintain a sterile body, it has to be colonized with some organisms, it is good if colonized with a less aggressive ones, we call them commensals. In special situations these commensals also can produce invasive infections. We are having a fairly good success with infections and its control and sharing our understanding with infections as a whole. A few activities of ours are the reason for the success, they are,

1. Examining the throat with tongue depressor of any child with fever or any signs of infection (would have examined close to 100,000 throats)

2. Taking throat swab for culture and sensitivity whenever there is a throat infection.

3. Aiming for complete cure of infection, whatever may be the antibiotic needed to control it, rather than going for symptomatic cure.

A child inside mother's uterus can be called sterile and the moment child is born it is exposed into the forest of organisms. It is then a fight between organisms to colonize the baby's skin, throat, gastrointestinal tract, genitalia etc. The colonized organism varies depending on the environment through which child was born (Vaginal delivery, LSCS), environment in which child was born (Labor room, NICU) and the environment in which child spends time with (mother, hospital room, house environment, any c/c infection in siblings, family members etc.), the material and substances child was exposed to (the water, oil, cloths they use) all are important in the initial colonization. Within days whole body and cavities are colonized. Usually, these colonizing organisms won't produce invasive diseases unless there are breaches in the primary barriers or the organism colonizing is highly virulent. Less virulent organism need breach in primary mucosal or skin barriers to enter. But highly virulent organisms make its own path into the system. Less virulent organisms more often tend to remain as commensals. We advise child to spend much of the time with the mother as there is more chance for the mother's skin organism to get colonized on the baby. Mother already would have antibody against her colonized organisms and baby will have all these antibodies transferred in-utero and also through breastmilk. So, the baby is protected from these organisms and are unlikely to get invasive infection. More antibodies reach the baby continuously through the breast milk, it is mainly IgA and IgG antibodies ready to protect the GIT and the blood stream. It is important for the mother to handle her baby the most, Kangaroo mother care (KMC) is a good method to promote this colonization. If the baby gets any pathogenic organism or more virulent organisms there is more chance for the baby to fall sick.

Once a baby gets infection it can behave in "n" number of ways. The response is different in invasive infection and non-invasive infections and is given in the following table.

**Table: 1** Type of infections and disease patterns.

| Type of infection | Method of entry / colonization | Disease patterns and end result |
|---|---|---|
| Invasive organism (highly virulent) | Highly invasive organisms can make their own pathway into the blood stream. | In invasive disease, either child succeeds or the organism succeeds. There is no chronic carrier state in invasive disease. But these organisms can get colonized in the GIT, oral cavity or on the skin. |
| Invasive organism (less virulent) | Entry after breach in primary barriers like skin and mucosa, through skin abrasions, mucosal injury or through inoculations. | Produces invasive diseases and there is no chronic carrier state in invasive diseases. But these organisms can get colonized in the GIT, oral cavity or on the skin. |
| Commensal organisms | Enter through breach in primary skin or mucosal barriers, or when they are highly immunocompromised. (immunocompromised state can occur when a child is very sick or in shock, when these commensals can also enter the blood stream) | Less likely to produce invasive diseases unless the child is highly immune compromised. Child usually have antibodies against commensal organisms. |

**Table: 2** Different types of attack on the baby.

| Type of attack on the baby | Results | Interpretation |
|---|---|---|
| Commensal organism producing infection (eg: CONS) | Less dramatic, as circulating antibody already present | Less dramatic infection |
| Chronically colonized virulent organism now becomes invasive (eg: staph aureus) | Since circulating antibodies are present disease can be less aggressive. | Less dramatic infection |
| New virulent* organism invading directly (eg: klebsiella) | Disease produced will be very aggressive because there are no antibodies to protect. | More severe infection needs good external help to contain. |
| New virulent organism colonizing and later invading | Invasion will be less aggressive as circulating antibodies will be there to defend. | As the organism is more virulent infection can be more severe even though circulating antibodies are present. |

\* virulency is produced by several factors

Now let us discuss what happens after an organism gets colonized in the body. All organism whatever may be their virulence, their ultimate aim is to multiply unrestrictedly, either outside or inside the body, all the other effects are a byproduct of this multiplication. Our body and other microorganisms try to prevent or suppress this multiplication and tries to eliminate the organism from the system.

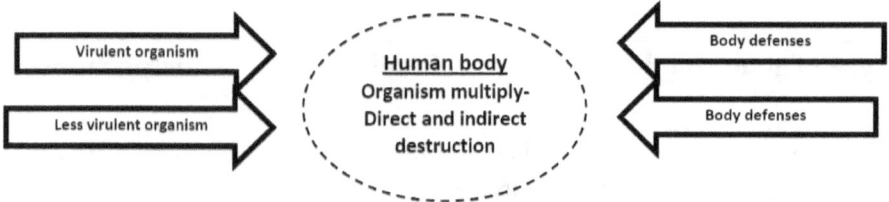

**Figure: 1** Organism and its interaction with human body

Organism itself and its metabolic products produce tissue and organ destruction. Body's defenses through immune mechanisms also produce tissue destruction. Newborn baby's immune system is immature and so there will be difficulty in detection of organisms, mounting an immune response and elimination of the organisms. All types of organisms whether commensal or virulent strains once inside produces bodily harm. No organism is innocent inside the body. The difference is in the nature of invasiveness and types of endotoxin production. For NICU baby organism gets entry through inoculation (IV fluid, IV canulation and other procedures), through colonization of oropharyngeal mucosa.

In pediatric age group the mechanism of entry is slightly different. There are only 5 entry point for any organisms to enter into the body. Entry can be through oro-naso pharyngeal tract, eyes, ears, anus and through urethral canal. It is obvious that only oro-naso-pharyngeal entry is important and organism entering through these reaches tonsillar and other lymphoid tissues, some are swallowed and reaches gastrointestinal tract, some try to enter respiratory tract. Organism reaching lymphoid tissue enter blood stream through lymph and produce fever and other symptoms. If it is an already exposed organism the organism gets eliminated in a few days by the circulating antibodies. Simultaneously body mounts an immune response with a time lag which differs from organism to organism and also depending on the history of previous exposures. There is a time lag for mounting an immune response through circulating antibodies. Organism-destroying immune cells (cytotoxic cells) are also activated (lymphocytes, monocytes, neutrophiles, N-K cells). Already existing antibodies in the blood may not be enough to neutralize the organisms immediately if the inoculum is large. Formed antibody and antigen combine to produce antigen-antibody complex which get deposited in the capillary bed which are chemoattractant and attract immune cells, which on activation produces symptoms like, local rise in temperature, rashes, itching, erythema etc. As the infection with the same organism (recurrent infection, a/c on c/c exacerbations) repeats the time for antibody response comes down and rash becomes earlier. Whenever there is Ag-Ab complexes immune cells are attracted and different types of rashes appear that can be fine, maculo-papular or urticarial in nature.

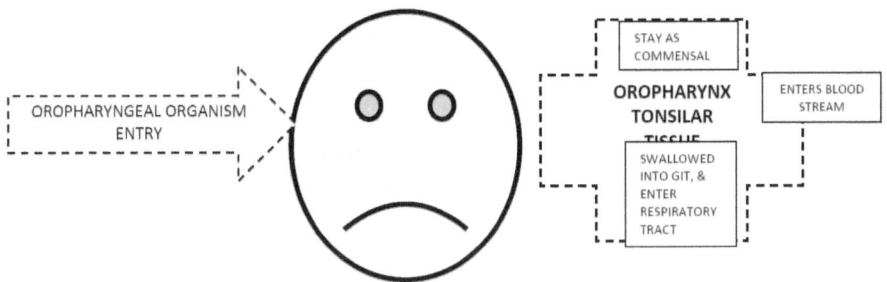

**Figure: 2**  Fate of organism after entry through mouth

In children invaded organisms are eliminated over a week, those entering and remaining inside the lymphoid tissue surrounding the oro-naso-pharyx takes different routes, they can be,

- Organism remains there as chronic carrier state self-protected from bodies defenses (secreting mucoid slimy layer) (less virulent organisms, commensal organisms)

- Some are completely eliminated from lymphoid tissue by the bodies defenses – this can happen if the tonsillar tissues are not chronically hypertrophied)
- Some are completely eliminated from the lymphoid tissue with the help of appropriate antibiotics in adequate doses for sufficient duration.
- Some produce invasive disease where organism is not eliminated by the bodies defense mechanisms and child falls sick and needs external help in the form of IV or oral antibiotics.

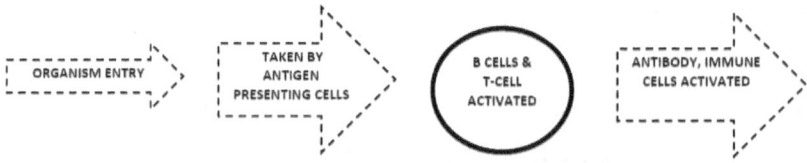

**Figure: 3** Immune response by body

Difference in Commensal & Less Aggressive Organisms

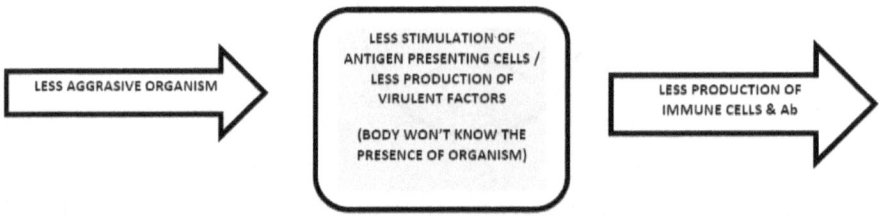

**Figure: 4** Immune response by body against less virulent organisms

## What are the bodies defenses against an organism invasion?

1. Bodies epithelial cells increases mucoid secretions in which organism gets trapped and are washed away.

2. Vomiting is a defense to quickly eliminate swallowed organism reaching stomach

3. Oro-nasal mucosal sensitivity increases, there is sneezing, coughing, hyperemia, congestion and increased blood supply. Immune cells reach submucosal area, immune mediators are released, mast cell degranulation to antigenic stimuli occurs. Nerves are more sensitized, allergic tendency appears, and cold exposure, dust exposure triggers sneezing and increased secretions, all these are to eliminate the organisms.

4. In the lymphoid tissue organisms come into contact with immune cells they destroy the organisms and take up specific antigen moieties and present it to antigen presenting cells to mount an immune response. They trigger B-cell and T-cells lines for activating humoral and cell mediated immune response respectively. After a lag the body produces an exaggerated immune response corresponding with that fever comes down, immune rashes appear. This shows that body has mounted and immune response and contained infection.

5. Organism getting inside the stomach are killed by the highly acidic environment.

6. Organism entering the respiratory tract are also eliminated through cough and by the action of ciliary beating. Some organisms paralyze the ciliary beating like that occurring in diphtheria infections so that their elimination is impaired.

7. Some organisms are permanently settled inside the lymphoid tissue (tonsil) protected from bodies defense mechanisms, this organism has to exhibit less virulence to escape immune surveillance. Our body increases its defense against these organisms through lymphoid hypertrophy. Organisms attempts several tricks to fool our body defenses. `

# Re-infections, Recurrent infections, Incompletely treated infections & Chronic infections

We have to clearly differentiate between re-infections, recurrent infections and incompletely treated infections, chronic infections and carrier state.

**Table: 1** Types of Infections and Definitions

| Type of infections | Definition | Cause and actions |
|---|---|---|
| Re-infection | Getting infection again and again from the same source | Getting infection from a family carrier, infected food source repeatedly (contaminated weaning food) |
| Recurrent infection | Getting infection again and again, source can be different or same | Getting infection again and again from same or different source. |
| Incompletely treated infections | Incompletely cured primary infection only to reappearing later | Infection treated but not cured fully, major symptoms may have subsided like, fever or cough, but not the primary focus of infection. |
| Chronic infections | Continuous infection with intermittent exacerbations | Major focus of infection persisting with reduced symptoms, with intermittent exacerbations. (eg. chronic URI) |

| Type of infections | Definition | Cause and actions |
|---|---|---|
| Carrier state | Continuous carriage of infection causing organism without much symptoms, but can spread to others and sometimes producing symptoms for themselves. We all are carriers of commensal organism, carrier becomes important when it is a pathogenic organism or MRD or MRSA | Focus of infection still persisting with no external symptoms, but show signs on examination. Carrier state is very common in URI. |
| Complete cure | No symptoms and signs and no trace of infection on examination | In case of URI, throat examination shows an absolutely normal throat. |

## Reinfections, recurrent infections and incompletely treated infections:

Both re-infections and recurrent infections are common in our community, we must be able to differentiate both clearly and find out the cause for each of these. Infections in the child hood have many longstanding implications than that occurring during adulthood. As child cannot express completely their complaints, it is the ability of parents and treating doctors which prompt treatment, many a times ending up in incomplete treatment. Some symptoms are dramatic and are forced to take urgent treatment, like for example fever, vomiting etc. Mild cough and mild abdominal discomfort are unattended. This also depends to some extend on the sensitivity of parents towards disease.

## CLINICAL SCENARIO

### Case: 1.

A 5-month-old child presented with fever and cough of 3 days duration, consulted a doctor gets treatment for 5 days and was symptom free. After 2 weeks child again gets fever and cold. This can be a case of reinfection from the same source. In reinfection the source is same, getting repeated infection from the same source. This can be from a family carrier or some food source which child was taking regularly. Unless you find out the source and remove it, child will get repeated infections. Complete cure of primary infection and removal of the source are both important for complete and permanent cure.

### Case: 2.

A 5-month-old child presented with fever and cough of 3 days duration, consulted a doctor gets treatment for 5 days and was relatively symptom free. After 5 days again presents with cough and cold, this can be a case of **incompletely treated primary infection**. If primary infection is not cured it creates different problems and have long term consequences. I can produce an endless list of problems produced by incompletely treated primary infections.

1. It can produce recurrent infections and its problems
2. Produce symptoms of nausea, vomiting, abdominal discomfort and abdominal bloating.
3. Constipation or intermittent loose motion (altered bowel habits).
4. Loss of appetite for the child due to infected secretions filling the stomach and also due to the tendency of nausea and vomiting.
5. Intermittent abdominal pain.

6. Disturbed sleep due to night time nasal block (temperature falls at night), cough and snoring.

7. Under weight and sometimes even stunting (whenever you see an underweight child have a look into the throat with tongue depressor)

8. Frequent rashes on face and limbs, more incidence of pyoderma

9. Fussy and irritable child because of constant irritation.

10. Continuous nasal discharge and ugly face.

11. Increased frequency of UTI and ASOM etc.

12. More signs of nutritional deficiencies seen because of decreased intake.

13. Spreads infections to sibling and rotation of infection between them happens

14. In children who are prone for wheezing with each episode of infections, these children will have recurrent wheezing episodes. If you treat the primary focus of infection the wheezing episodes becomes a rarity.

15. Frequent headaches and even taking treatment for migraine (headache and vomiting). These children feel better after vomiting because of relief from dumping all the accumulated stomach secretions, so may mimic symptoms of migraine. Seen several cases treated falsely with migraine medications.

The list is endless and so never leave an upper respiratory tract infection untreated simply because it is less discomforting. If you try to co-relate with any listed symptoms with URTI then we will be forced to cure the infection completely. I always look into a child's throat with a tongue depressor, whenever a child comes with any of the mentioned symptoms and if required take a throat swab for culture and sensitivity. This I have been doing for the last 13 years and seen more than 100,000 throats and done more than 10,000 of throat cultures. So, I have a fair idea about the type of organisms and its resistance patterns and type of manifestations. Multiple organisms are very common and if infections are not going away you have to attack both the strains simultaneously. Multiple organisms are usually gram positive and gram negative and less likely to have two organisms from the same class, but possible, seen cases of E-coli and klebsiella cultures from the same swab. (One has to be familiar with normal throat patterns to identify subtle variations seen in abnormal throats)

## CHRONIC INFECTION.

Some children and adults carry infection in their throat for long duration sometimes even for years. They experience periodic exacerbations of cough cold and or wheezing with constant hypersensitivity to dust and cold exposure. Invariably they are labeled as "allergic" and will be on several allergic medications. They have symptoms of stuffy nose sneezing occasional cough. The problem with them are they are never disease free any time and they harbor MDR organisms and spreads infection to their contacts. Children are highly prone to this spread. Children having chronic infections are also similar with congested throat and they get exacerbations very easily with cold exposure or intake of some citrus fruits etc. The organisms residing (throat swab C&S) are usually resistant to commonly used antibiotics. Take a throat swab and find the culprit and treat completely. Seen several cases of MRSA colonization in parents whose children are having chronic URTI. Once you treat these chronic infections completely their appetite improves, they get better sleep, growth picks up, less absenteeism, less wheezing attacks etc.

## CARRIER STATE

Carrier state persons are having less episodes of exacerbations and are relatively symptom free compared to chronically infected people. Only a very detailed history taken can expose a carrier state of MDR organism or MRSA. We all are commensal organism carriers and become problematic only when you carry a pathogenic organism, MDR or MRSA. Identifying a carrier is important to prevent repeated spread of infection to kids.

In summary infection should be treated completely. Upper respiratory tract infections are the one which are prone for chronicity silently. A chronic CSOM is obvious and we are forced to take treatment completely. Similarly, a chronic urinary tract infection is less likely because most of the UTI are completely treated in the acute stage itself.

## Chapter 29

# INDIAN "JUGAAD" WAY OF "NO- EXTRA COST" SAFE COOLING FOR HIE

Our NICU is a 12 bedded ICU and we get approximately 4 to 5 cases of birth asphyxia cases per year for cooling therapy. As the case load is low, we cannot afford expensive cooling machines which cost approximately 15 to 20 lakhs. Over the years we have successfully treated more than 15 cases of birth asphyxia. We do it with simple coolant packs and ordinary air conditioning system. We don't have any problem in maintaining the rectal temperature in the recommended range, the fluctuations are also minimal. We started this with lots of apprehension and we are now confidently doing it. No extra machines are needed as all NICU's are having air conditioning units and only thing needed is courage for doing this. In the entire district only one cooling system is available and with upward cost of 15 lakh it is not affordable in most NICUs. The following is the method we follow.

1. As soon as birth asphyxia case referral is informed, **coolant pack** (2 pack) (used to send medication/ vaccines from distributors to pharmacy, freely available with pharmacy) (not ice pack) is taken from refrigerator and rapped thickly in a cloth and kept ready in the fridge. By wrapping in thick cloth cover the cold injury is nonexistent.

2. For cooling purpose, a separate room (small to medium sized) with air conditioning system (1 ton or 1-1/2 ton) is preferred.

3. Follow all the standard protocols recommended for cooling like, neuro examination schedules, investigations, temperature monitoring, rewarming etc.

4. Bed is kept ready,

    a. Switch off the warmer

    b. Monitors, rectal temperature probe all are kept ready

    c. Ventilator, intubation equipments are kept ready

    d. As soon as the baby comes, vitals are measured, rectal temperature probe secured properly,

    e. Make sure shock is corrected with normal saline and inotropes.

    f. If no severe shock, coolant wrapped in thick cloth is place behind the back side. You can change the position of the pack but that is not necessary (cold injury is not seen, but if you use ice packs there are chances for injury. During melting of ice lots of heat is used at a faster pace than coolant packs, so there can be more injury with ice packs. Coolant packs takes up heat more slowly and in a controlled manner).

    g. Air conditioning temperature can be set at 20-24*C and adjusted according to your environmental condition and baby's rectal temperature.

    h. Rectal temperature probe is placed properly (5cm inside). Display a notice stating the set rectal temperature required (desired rectal temperature: 33 ±5*C) so that everyone is aware of the target temperature.

    i. If required intubated and ventilated

j.  UVC and UAC lines are inserted and blood collected for blood gas measurements, all other investigations send.

k.  Shock and metabolic acidosis are aggressively managed.

5. Higher antibiotics may be required, very baseline antibiotics (ampicillin & gentamycin) can result in cooling failure. This is because of the highly suppressed immunity in the cooling baby. Shock and sepsis are the major factors of cooling failure.

6. Uncontrolled shock is the one which forces us to terminate the cooling and shock is mostly due to infections.

7. Place the coolant packs at different sites, monitor temperature continuously once the temperature nears the cooling range remove the coolant packs. After that usually temperature can be maintained with air-conditioning alone. Once the desired temperature is reached then the maintenance of temperature is fairly easy. If the rectal temperature dips lower warmer can be switched on.

8. Sent investigations at regular intervals,

9. Seizure is aggressively controlled (seizures are less once cooling is initiated).

The is the method we follow and is very successful and no real preparations are needed to cool a baby. It is now just like any other routine to cool a baby in our NICU, no extra arrangements are needed. Twice we had to abundant cooling and that was due to uncontrolled shock and sepsis. Temperature maintenance was never a problem. There was no skin injury and the need for placement of coolant pack repeatedly was also very less. The temperature maintenance was surprisingly excellent and easy. The fluctuations in baby's rectal temperature are surprisingly less. Many units may be using this simple method, writing this to give encouragement and confidence for others to follow. This will result in the reduction of price of the cooling equipment.

By this method there is no extra cost incurred, every neonatal setup can start this. There is no time delay in starting cooling, only problem is your neonatal care should be excellent otherwise failure due to other causes can occur. It is not advisable to attempt cooling the baby if your NICU is ill equipped to handle critical cases.

We also use cooling for neonatal status epilepticus with excellent results. Babies only rarely have seizures after starting cooling. The number of anticonvulsants used are also less. The outcome is excellent as there is less brain damage from seizures. We give cooling for seizures babies for 1-3 days.

**Advantages of this low-cost cooling**

- No extra cost involved.
- Can start immediately without any delay
- Any unit can start this method
- Hurry burry of transferring the baby is avoided, so also infections
- Can avoid costly equipments
- We can also use this methods to control resistant seizures.
- Any unit practicing level -2 neonatal care confidently can try this method.

Anybody trying this method of cooling should have utmost care of babies with close temperature monitoring especially when keeping cool packs, unattended cool packs result in baby going into dangerous hypothermia. Since there are no equipment involved in monitoring the nurses are the eye and ears of the baby.

# Chapter 30

# IS INCOMPLETELY TREATED URTI THE MAIN CAUSE OF COMMUNITY SPREAD AND DISEASE BURDEN IN THE COMMUNITY?

The upper respiratory tract infection (URTI) is the most common (>90%) infection encountered in the OPD and most of my discussions revolves around URI. Standard text books never discuss about this common infection in detail as it is taken for granted that everybody knows about this and need not waste time discussing it, but nobody realizes that it causes 90% of the disease burden in the community. If you do a cross sectional study in the community you can see various types of infections, some are acute infections, some are in convalescent stage, some cured and some incompletely treated and going into the chronic phase. Of these the one going into the chronic phase is the dangerous group as they are the one maintaining spread in the community. Chronic infections can be,

- Asymptomatic
- Asymptomatic with intermittent exacerbations
- Symptomatic with intermittent exacerbations

Asymptomatic variety escapes detection but spreads in the family to the other siblings and other family members. They can have subtle other symptoms like occasional vomiting, loss of appetite, undernutrition, constipation, etc. If you look into the throat with a tongue depressor you can see the inflamed tonsillo-pharyngeal tissue. Some doctors can corelate the symptoms with this chronic infection, some don't. If the organism present is a resistant variety, then he or she spreads this resistant variety in the community. Always do a throat swab culture and sensitivity to know the nature of organisms.

Over the months with each exacerbations the chronic variety undergo exposure to different varieties of antibiotics and the organism residing can become resistant to antibiotics. These organisms can have acquired resistant to commonly used antibiotics like amoxicillin, azithromycin, second generation cephalosporines etc. If we don't stop it spread these resistant organisms will spread. Usually, these chronic carriers are labelled as "allergic" individuals because of the upper respiratory tract hypersensitivity due to the infection. There is a new trend in the community for treating these chronic carriers as "allergic individuals" and treat symptomatically with inhalers and montelukast, without searching for the root cause of this "allergy". Let's us discuss this topic in detail.

## A CASE STUDY:

An 8-month-old male child presented with high fever, cold, nasal block, vomiting and abdominal distention of 3 days duration. A throat examination with tongue depressor was done and found out that throat and pharynx were congested, swollen and red. A diagnosis of acute upper respiratory tract infection (URTI) was made. Child was treated with decongestive measures, antipyretics, antiemetics, nasal drops and started on oral antibiotic Augmentin. Child became afebrile and was better and reviewed again on day 5, at that time child only had mild symptoms of cold and doctor reassured the parents and he stopped oral antibiotics and asked to continued decongestants for 3 more days. A repeat throat examination was not done. Child was doing well as most symptoms disappeared except for mild nasal stuffiness in the morning and mild abdominal distention. Two months after this incident this child came to my OPD with complains of intermittent cry, mild abdominal distension, nasal stuffiness, occasional vomiting especially after feeds or in the morning for the last 3-4 weeks. No fever or cough, child was growing well. Usual tendency is to treat this as separate new infection.

I took a detailed history and asked specifically when these symptoms started and mother told me that all these symptoms aggravated for the last 3-4 weeks but actually everything started from the URI 2 months back. Immediately I got the diagnosis and examined the throat and took a throat swab for culture and sensitivity. Throat was congested, tonsil moderately enlarged, covered with mucoid secretions. This is a clear-cut case of incompletely treated first attack of URI 2 months back. I made a diagnosis of acute on chronic tonsillopharyngitis. Most doctors without realizing this starts on another course of same antibiotics (Augmentin/ Amoxicillin) and organism is most likely to be resistant to these antibiotics because these organisms had survived a course of Augmentin already. But no fault in repeating a course of Augment for this child provided you do a repeated throat examination and see for the complete cure and if not, go for a higher antibiotic according to culture and sensitivity report. There is a natural selection process happening with each course of incomplete treatment. In this case you need to definitely take a throat swab and start on a higher antibiotic like cefuroxime.

## PITFALLS IN TREATMENT

- Wrong diagnosis, wrong interpretation.
- Incomplete treatment (doctor or patient stops prematurely)
- Inappropriate antibiotic choice.
- Insufficient dose (insufficient calculated dose & children spills and vomits drugs).
- Insufficient duration.

- Incomplete internal cure with improvement of external symptoms (mother will be happy but you should not be happy until and unless you reach complete cure -internally & externally).

I started on the following: (Aim is to decrease symptoms and complete cure)

- Decongestive measures (to decrease the secretions and discomfort to the child)
- Oxymetazoline (to decrease nasal stuffiness and the number of secretions, normal saline only decreases the thickness of secretions, can be ok for mild symptoms)
- Next line antibiotics (Cefuroxime)
- Take throat swab for culture and sensitivity.
- Review after 5-7 days (according to the level of sickness) and see the throat and ask for the relief from symptoms)
- Change antibiotics, if required based on C & S report and condition of throat and decide on duration of treatment
- If required ask for one or two revisits, don't hesitate to upgrade antibiotics.
- Then you can add an montelukast for 3 to 6 weeks for suppressing flaring of recurrent of infections and to decrease the size of tonsil as there are some signs of chronic tonsilitis.
- Ask to avoid cold drinks (cold water, ice cream), citrus fruits, watermelon etc. as these can cause flaring up of infection.

**Culture and sensitivity report came as:** Smear showing GPC, GNB with culture growing E-Coli resistant to amoxycillin + clavulanic acid and azithromycin, sensitive to aminoglycoside, ofloxacin, meropenem and moderately sensitive to cefuroxime. It is actually a mixed infection, both gram positive and gram-negative organisms were seen. This is a highly debatable topic but for me a practical approach had paid dividends for my patients. In this case you need to treat E-Coli with appropriate antibiotics. No need to do repeat throat swab, but definitely do repeated throat examination with a tongue depressor.

The same case can present with the following combinations of organisms (same symptoms but can have different organism).

- GPC, – Penicillin resistant streptococci or staph aureus (MSSA)
- GPC, – MRSA or MRSE
- GPC, GNB, – MRSA & MDR Klebsiella
- GPC, GNB – MRSA & PDR Pseudomonas
- GNB, – PDR pseudomonas sensitive only to polymyxin-B.
- GNB, – E-Coli, highly resistant, only sensitive to meropenem, tigecycline and polymyxin

All these kinds of organisms have been encountered, as a clinician you should be able to treat these cases properly without labelling these as chronic allergic patients. From my experience if you treat these properly all these allergic symptoms vanishes. Once these kinds of organisms get into your throat, they settle there for long durations and produce mild cough, sneezing, running nose, with intermittent exacerbations (URI or wheezing) and will have all the signs of allergy, and are highly prone to be labelled as allergic. These kinds of cases are usually labelled as allergic, most family members would be carrying these organisms from internal spread. So, I am highly skeptical of the diagnosis of allergy, see the chapter on allergy for my completely different view on allergy.

**Always do a throat examination, sent a throat swab for C&S, treat completely. Not only aim for cure of external symptoms but also aim for internal cure.** (Most Microbiologist has a tendency to report all commonly seen oral pathogens as commensals, ask them to report what they see and leave the interpretation to the treating doctors).

**CASE DISCUSSION:**

**This is a typical case of chronic infection following an incompletely treated primary infection. What are the faults done during treatment of primary infection?**

- Repeat throat examination on second visit was not done to make sure infection was completely cured or not.

- Doctor mainly took external symptoms (fever cough vomiting etc.) as a guide for treatment (stopped treatment when fever, vomiting, cough subsided). He didn't make sure whether the primary infection which caused all these symptoms had completely gone or not. This is possible only through a repeat throat examination. (this same thing can happen if you treat fever symptoms of UTI without doing repeated urine RE examination at the end).

- A throat swab for culture was not done neither during the first visit or subsequently when mild symptoms was persisting. By not doing this we don't know whom we are fighting with.

- This is the common way of converting a primary episode of infection into a chronic problem lasting for years.

**How to treat the above case properly.**

- Always examine the throat, send throat swab for culture whenever seems necessary, (send when there is resistance for complete cure).

- Give decongestants, xylometazoline nasal drops, colic aid drops, antibiotics (appropriate). This is for symptomatic relief especially important for small babies.

- Chose antibiotics according to culture and sensitivity, if not available gradually step-up antibiotics and see for the full cure.
- Treat instigating cause like oil bath (oil is a good medium for bacterial growth), treat the carriers of infection properly (mother or any other care givers), check for cleanliness of weaning foods etc.
- Repeated throat examination, aim for complete cure of primary infection and don't just aim for symptomatic relief.

**Our disease burden and spread in the community is mainly due to incompletely treated chronic infections**

From my experience I have learned that our disease burden in the community and spread is mainly due to the incompletely treated infections. I always aim for the complete cure for all variety of infections may it be throat infections, UTI, ear infections, skin infections. I also try to find the source of recurrence of infections and give advice for that. Always try to find out and treat other carriers.

**Steps in treating chronic upper respiratory tract infection.**

- Try to find the status of infection by looking inside the throat with tongue depressor.
- Take throat swab for C&S
- Start with 2nd level antibiotics and see the response, with each visit see throat properly for cure.
- Change to culture report-based antibiotics, if seems appropriate, don't 100% blindly follow the culture report, it can sometimes be misleading. These are only act as a guide post, you are the decision maker. Sometimes response will exactly follow the culture and sensitivity reports.
- Identify other carriers and treat (siblings, father, mother or grandparents etc.)

- Other source of infections, from food, from pica, oil application, bad quality well water (ask for the type of septic tank and its distance from the well, they may be boiling water for drinking, but organism can enter the body during bathing with bad well water and produce symptoms of cold first then other symptoms. Well water may contain resistant E-coli. (Test well water for C & S.)

- Can add Montelukast for 1 to 2 months to prevent flair up of infections later and to decrease the inflammation of chronic tonsilitis.

- Treat each flair of infections appropriately and if everything is going well child becomes better and symptom free intervals increases and each episode becomes less and less intense.

- Tips to decrease the flair up of infections. Avoid cold exposure (ice cream, cold water, juice), try to avoid or decrease consumption of citrus fruits, watermelon, grapes etc. These can flare up the already existing infections or superadd another infection depending on the contamination of the food consumed.

## How is chronic carriers act as spreaders?

A chronic carrier can be an adult or a child. Child spreads the infection to siblings or other children in the neighborhood, to the other children at school. Those who are exposed manifests in different ways, some will have active infection and may be forced to take treatment, minority of group can become silent carriers and majority will not have any symptoms. More symptomatic patients will get treated and mild infections are treated conservatively. Carrier subgroup of patients may again act as spreaders. During covid-19 pandemic due to the extensive use of mask, hand sanitizer, lack of contact and closed schools has dramatically decreased the incidence of infections and wheezing in children. Hundreds of children labelled as allergic on inhalers and steroids didn't need any of the medications for over one year, how is that possible. Severe infections and admissions have also dramatically decreased. It is because each episodes of exaggeration have infections as a trigger (viral or bacterial) and under treated infections remains inside the child. There is also exacerbations of wheezing and infections during lunar variations.

Chronic spreaders are usually labeled as allergic persons, because of recurrent allergic symptoms upon exposure to dust and cold. Upon exposure they start to sneeze or start to cough but won't take proper treatment as their symptoms subside in a weeks' time without much treatment or using some local remedies. If you ask specifically, they may say they have occasional cough or cough especially in the morning hours. I have done throat swab on these chronic carriers and on several occasions turn out to be MDR organisms or MRSA.

It is generally assumed that mild symptoms mean common sensitive organisms and very dramatic symptoms means very dangerous organisms. This is not true because a MRSA carrier can produce very mild and indolent symptoms and escape treatment with occasional exacerbations. A sensitive streptococcus into a vulnerable person can produce high fever and sickness. Only from response to the given antibiotics gives us a clue to the nature of antibiotic resistance. Both sensitive and resistant organisms can produce mild as well as very severe infections, it mainly depends on the precipitating factors and vulnerability. Precipitating factors can be preceding viral infections and damage to the epithelium. Most children upon reaching a tertiary center would have received 2-3 variety of antibiotics that means we are dealing with an organism which are resistant to commonly used antibiotics. This is more so in case of chronic long-standing carriers, who would have exposed to several layers of treatment. Other mechanism of producing chronic carriers is by the usage of substandard antibiotics or usage of subclinical dosage and incomplete treatment by prematurely stopping antibiotics either by doctor or by patient. Other known method is through natural selection, where by the sensitive organism dies and resistant organism survives. So, with each incomplete treatment more and more resistant organisms will survive and they become the majority. This natural selection can happen when there are multiple types of organism whereby a particular group will survive the antibiotic on slot or helps in selective growth of resistant brood of organisms.

Inside a family spread of infection is fast especially between father, mother and siblings. Any organism can spread from anywhere to any areas especially between sexually active partners.

**Mother or father any area infection (URI, UTI) can reach as URI in a breastfeeding child.**

Chronic carrier → siblings → spread to other children in play group → spread in school → other kid's infection taken to other family members or kids → some become chronic carriers → this cycle thrives.

This cycle would have stopped if we have used and treated primary case with appropriate antibiotics even if using higher antibiotics (even using ofloxacin, clarithromycin, or even IV antibiotics). Nowadays these chronic cases are treated with inhalers and are labelled as "allergic" persons. "Allergy" is a widely misused term.

One important point is to identify the exact source of recurrent infections. There are many causes with regional variations depending on the cultural practices but listing few of the prominent ones observed during my practice. Listing causes starting from birth onwards.

1. **From hospital colonization after deliver:** this is a prominent cause if you get colonized by a pathologic organism like Klebsiella, E-Coli, Acinetobacter, MRSA, MRSE etc. This is especially true if there is any NICU stay for long, colonization

from improperly maintained labor room, resuscitation table etc. They can have varied symptoms starting from newborn period to varying periods as long as 6 months to one year or more. Those coming to me are fully recognized (culture of throat) and treated. Symptoms varies from constant nasal block, feeding difficulty, nausea, vomiting, occasional cough, abdominal distension, seizure like up rolling due to mucus obstructing the throat and subsequent difficulty. (Child cannot spit out thick mucus nor can he swallow thick mucus voluntarily, struggles with up rolling of eyes). Seen several cases landing up in OPD as "?seizures" I just do one throat examinations and prescribe medications to decrease secretions and use oxymetazoline nasal drops (not normal saline, it won't help here) and a "good" antibiotic, child and parents are happy.

These colonized organisms from NICU or hospital won't go by its own, they stay and produces exacerbations of varying degrees. Already they have circulating antibodies against them so highly invasive diseases are less likely.

2. Any infect family members (including sibling can spread infection)

3. Ceremonies like 28th day function in Hindu families, Mamodisa in Christian families, hair removal function in Muslim families are point of source for infection. In relation to these they can give holy water, Vyambu, Bhrami, rubbed gold water etc. All are a potential source of infections, as lots of people gather for these functions.

4. Mother taking ayurvedic medications post delivery is a common practice and can upset child's abdomen and induce colic, nausea vomiting and even loose motion or constipation.

5. Any weaning food ill prepared is a source of infection.

6. Some fruits are prone for infection especially available in our country, they are grapes ( they are fully exposed throughout transport and dust and flies are a common seen, more over pesticide use is excessive). Watermelon is also a source of infection, several children come to me with fever and cough and cold after taking this. My theory is like this, since watermelon is big after cutting half goes into fridge for later use, this is the part which causes problem. Inside of fridge is a highly potential source of infection except inside freezer. Organisms can grow rampantly outside freezer compartment (temp: 2-8* C). In families the inside cleaning of fridge is a rarity and lots of food and vegetables are stuffed and fridge is highly colonized. Anything coming out is infectious. Other infectious fruits are mango (brought from outside, same as grapes).

7. Another potential but hidden source is contaminated well water. Well water can get contaminated from nearby septic tanks. See the type of septic tank and the distance from it. We do culture of well water in our lab and seen unhygienic growth of coliforms and advise periodic Potassium Permanganate treatment of well water which is freely available from health authorities. One defense by parents is that they never give un-boiled water to their children. Organism usually enter through bathing as they never boil the water, they only make it warm.

8. Another common source of infection is from oil application to the babies. Oil application and massage is a good traditional practice please discontinue that if your child is getting frequent URTIs because your oil can be the culprit. In Kerala most people use coconut oil, this can be a good

medium for the organism to growth. If you keep a small quantity of coconut oil in a vessel for few days it's smell and texture changes due to the growth of organism, if you apply it over the baby what to expect? So, we advise to warm up the oil at regular intervals.

9. From asymptomatic or symptomatic carriers in the family.

10. From playschool or school.

11. From playing in mud or dust, but children has to play in these to get resistance from these, body has to process these potential allergen in the early ages to make them tolerant, otherwise lots of real allergy can be expected in later life.

12. Habit of pica is a source of URTI

13. Sleeping in a fully closed room with several family members can produce repeated infection for the vulnerable. This produces rebreathing of air, humidity increases organism exchange can occur, morning they can feel tired (from $CO_2$ rebreathing) and with stuffy nose and sometimes with cough and cold.

14. From reusing uncleaned utensils.

15. From multivitamin medication contamination from dipping into the mouth of the baby and putting back the dropper into the bottle without cleaning and this medication bottle can act as a source.

Most of the above ways of getting infection result in URTI or GIT infection (both has the same entry point), the only way to establish infection is looking into the throat with a tongue depressor. Without tongue depressor you may miss most the infections unless large children cooperating well by saying "Ah" well. Looking into the throat can help you to establish infections in may circumstances. Here are some of the lists of circumstances where it may help.

1. For establishing a throat infection, tonsilitis, pharyngitis, adenoids etc.
2. Fever with or without a focus.
3. Vomiting, nausea
4. Not taking food or taking breastfeeding
5. Chronic allergy, sneezing, coughing, constant throat clearing
6. Bad breath
7. Chronic or acute abdominal pain
8. Under nutrition
9. Constipation or loose motion
10. Incessant cry in a newborn, not sleeping at night, occasional cough, nasal block etc.
11. Excessive abdominal distension, abdominal bloating, abdominal discomfort, complaints of excessive gas.
12. Excessive oral secretions or drooling from mouth
13. Recurrent fever, infections, URTI etc.
14. Any PUO, rule out throat infections before proceeding forward, take throat swab for culture and sensitivity.
15. Child with PICA can have infection in throat.
16. Recurrent UTI, upper respiratory tract infection can be a primary focus for spread.
17. Excessive cheek rash in a newborn or few months old baby. Hidden throat infection with infected saliva causing rash where ever it comes into contact, which spreads to neck and

other parts of the body. Examine the throat properly and treat infection if there is one.

So, just by examining the throat with a tongue depressor you can remove several of the mysteries, my practice changed almost 14 years ago when I discovered this magic of throat examination. Then only you start to connect thing otherwise you are in the blind. During my practice the diagnosis of PUO is a rarity, occasionally some real PUO comes. Let this be a real help for those who are not examining the throat and an encouragement for those who are already practicing it.

# Chapter 31

# IS "ALLERGY" A SCAPEGOAT DIAGNOSIS?

Allergy is the most misused term seen in pediatric practice. Anything which is not properly explainable, recurrent, anything which sneezes, anything which wheezes, anything which itches, any skin with rash, all are grouped under allergy and treated accordingly. It is acting like an excuse diagnosis. Everything is put in the allergy basket. Simple definition of allergy can be defined as a particular set of manifestation due to an exaggerated immune response against a particular trigger. So, there should be a trigger, exaggerated immune response and a wide variety of manifestations. Allergy word should only be given the importance as the word fever. Fever is just a symptom and it can be due to numerous causes, similarly allergy is just a manifestation and underlying cause we have to dig out. But what is happening is after labelling as allergy all efforts to find the basic underlying cause stops.

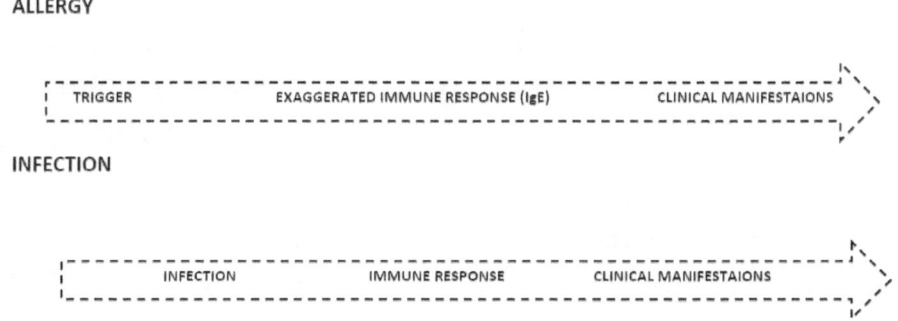

**Figure: 1** Allergy Vs Infection

{**Definition of allergy. (Nelson text 21ˢᵗ Ed)**

The term allergy represents the clinical expression of IgE -mediated allergic diseases that have a familial predisposition and that manifests as hypersensitivity in target organs such as the lungs, skin, gastrointestinal tract and nose. Allergic or atopic patients have an altered state of reactivity to common environmental food antigen that do not cause clinical reactions in unaffected people. Patients with clinical allergy usually produce immunoglobulin E (IgE) antibodies to the antigen that trigger their illness.}

Any infection also has the same consequence like that of allergy, the immune response is moderate and not exaggerated, clinical manifestations are also like that of allergy. In allergy we remove or avoid the trigger and thus decrease the recurrence of allergy. But in practice mostly the exact trigger is not known. When the infection is subclinical or chronic it is not recognized as infections and because of the similarity in clinical manifestations these infections are misdiagnosed as allergy and treated accordingly. This is what is happening in at least some cases of asthma, chronic URTI etc. From my experience numerous established cases of asthma has being cured of its recurrence simply by treating the underlying infections adequately. Why in a child with first episode of wheeze or recurrent episodes of wheezing we are forced to do investigations to rule out primary complex? It is because underlying primary complex can be a cause for this wheezing. Similarly, any chronic infection can be a central cause for wheezing.

There are hundreds of triggers which the body is exposed, but they don't end up in allergy. Immune system is constantly in fight with outside and inside world (self), but won't produce allergy. Incompletely treated infections with exacerbations can mimic an allergy, but in this case if you treat the infections properly the allergy disappears.

## Let us see the preparations body makes in case of an upper respiratory tract infections.

1. Lymphoid tissues around oro-pharyngeal areas are made more efficient: increases in size, increases in blood supply (redness), nerve ending becomes more sensitive to stimuli, immune cells migrate to this area in large numbers.

2. Nasopharyngeal areas become more sensitive; nerve ending is made more sensitive, only small trigger is needed for an exaggerated response.

3. Nasopharyngeal area become more hyperemic and more blood flows through these areas resulting in stuffy nose this is to trap organisms. Early morning nasal stuffiness, sneezing occurs.

4. There is increased secretion of mucus to trap organisms and expel it. This produces running nose.

5. All reflexes namely, sneezing reflex, cough reflex, nausea and vomiting reflexes are all exaggerated because of the sensitive nerve endings.

6. Nausea, vomiting and cough all are to expel the organisms to the outside.

7. Any infection anywhere can produce skin manifestations like erythema (vasodilation), fine rash, maculopapular rash, nodules, pustules (local infections), most of these rashes are due to deposition of immune complexes (Antigen-Antibody complexes) and activation of immune cells and its secondary reactions. Immune complexes are also deposited in the capillary beds of kidney and so also in all capillary beds. Can we call these immune complex depositions as allergy? The answer is no. For most new infections by day five immune complexes are formed and it results in the appearance of rash and fever usually subsides

after that as circulating organisms are all eliminated by circulating antibodies. It is unfortunate that these rashes are mistaken as allergic reaction to the antibiotic and there is a tendency to stop it, usual victim is the ampicillin group. With each recurrence of infection, the time interval to appearance of rash decreases and in chronic infection rash becomes constant.

8. When the infection becomes chronic all the mentioned systems get exaggerated or hypertrophied, like slight exposure to dust or cold makes the person to sneeze excessively. Sneezing reflex stimulates epithelial cells to secrete more, mast cell release etc. can occur.

9. Once antibodies are produced there is check on the bacteremia from local infections, local bacterial growth is also suppressed from circulating antibodies in secretions and in blood.

10. In chronic infections any trigger like cold exposure, superadded viral infections, any stress, trauma all can exacerbate the existing infections.

These are the various manifestations of an infection and that same infection becomes chronic all the actions are exaggerated and can mimic like allergy, but basically is just a chronic infection. The importance of this identification is, these "allergic type" manifestations disappear once the infections are removed. Rather than labelling everything that sneezes as allergy, try to separately identify each. Like allergy we have to try to eliminate the trigger, that is, infections. Differentiation between pure allergy (milk protein allergy, cow's milk allergy) and subclinical chronic infection should be made. The following are the types of allergic reactions existing.

**Four types of allergy are,** (type -1 is the type which is implicated in allergic diseases).

1. Type-1 or anaphylactic reactions mediated by IgE antibodies, cause release of histamine and other chemicals. Mast cell release occurs.
   - e.g.: asthma, allergic rhinitis, allergic dermatitis, food allergy, anaphylaxis (allergic shock).
2. Type-2 or cytotoxic reactions, mediated by IgG and IgM antibodies
   - e.g.: autoimmune hemolytic anemia, immune thrombocytopenia, autoimmune neutropenia.
3. Type-3 or Immunocomplex reactions, mediated by IgM and IgG antibodies, forms antigen-antibody complexes.
   - e.g. Lupus, serum sickness, arthus reaction.
4. Type -4 or Cell mediated reactions, delayed hypersensitivity, takes 48 to 72 hrs or longer to appear
   - e.g. Tuberculosis, fungal infections.

I have seen several cases of labelled asthma on prolonged steroid inhalation medications and oral medications suddenly becoming symptom free on properly treating the underlying infections. Here underlying infections were the trigger for asthmatic attacks. Immune reactions were suppressed with the help of medications. This current covid-19 pandemic is a live example of infection as the main trigger for asthma. After starting covid-lock down asthmatic attacks drastically came down. A simple mask can prevent all symptoms of asthma to subside, able to stop most of the medications. Then we can expect a campaign against face mask and its side effects in the near future ("mask induced lung diseases"!). My point is, always remove the infection component from all allergic diseases to get a clearer picture and a complete cure. This is good for the patient but not so good for pharma companies.

Everything that sneezes is not allergy, everything that wheezes is not allergy, any skin rash or itching is not allergy. Find the underlying cause and treat. Don't make allergy an scapegoat diagnosis.

# Chapter 32

# IS THERE ANY RELATIONSHIP BETWEEN SEIZURES AND VITAMIN D?

Febrile and nonfebrile seizures are a very commonly encountered problem in pediatric practice. It is also the most panicking condition encountered both for doctors and parents. If not properly managed it can end in ventilatory requirements and even death. Over the years of my carrier the incidence of febrile seizure has increased drastically. We have found an association (for the last 4 years) with low levels of vitamin D with febrile as well as nonfebrile seizures. We always do vitamin D estimation as part of panel of investigations for seizures. We have conducted a survey and found that >90% of children with febrile or nonfebrile seizures have low values of vitamin D levels on admission. Those who are presenting with status epilepticus invariably have very low levels of vitamin D levels.

As a treatment strategy we prescribe adequate doses of vitamin D supplementations as a preventive strategy to prevent recurrence of seizure. Seizure recurrence for our follow up babies is very less after vitamin D supplementation. More than that those who had status epilepticus rarely had any second recurrence of status epilepsy while on vitamin D supplementation and anticonvulsants. During my early years of practice, status epilepsy baby invariably had breakthrough seizures. Those babies diagnosed with channelopathies have recurrent seizures which are resistant to treatment as usual. All these shows a define role of vitamin D in the genesis of febrile and nonfebrile seizures. Simultaneous calcium levels are not always low with seizures, but mostly on the lower side of normal. On the preventive aspect it seems vitamin D supplementation is a better prophylaxis medication than any other drugs. We give vitamin D supplementation for 6 months minimum and advise them to increase sunlight exposure.

Since vitamin D is acting through the nuclear receptors, hundreds and hundreds of genes are activated and it is making some fundamental changes in the neurocircuitry of the brain in order to prevent recurrence of seizure. After giving vitamin D the chance for recurrence of seizure later even after stopping vitamin D is less, but the chance of recurrence increases for nonfebrile seizures. As I have discussed in another chapter vitamin D can instantly decrease the episodes of breath holding spells. Breath holding spells can also be considered a type of seizure. The incidence of benign sleep myoclonus is also seen less with the routine supplementation of vitamin D after birth.

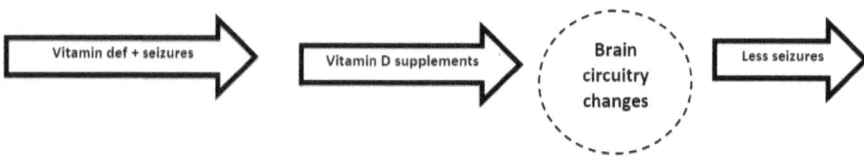

**Figure: 1** Vitamin D deficiency and seizures

**Points to remember and future suggestions:**

- Include vitamin D estimations as part of seizure panel.
- Start supplementing vitamin D and calcium as treatment and preventive strategy
- In future vitamin D supplementations may be included in the seizure prophylaxis
- Breath holding spells are easily controlled with vitamin D (breath holding spell can be considered as a type of seizure).

- Can take up studies to see the normalization of EEG with vitamin D alone, there are neurocircuitry changes happening with long term vitamin D supplementation. Moreover, good response is seen with vitamin D in cases of speech delay and developmental delay.

- Due to the complexity of action through genes vitamin D may not work as a drug during a seizure attack, rather it acts better as a prophylactic long-term medicine.

- I am not saying all seizures will cease to exist with vitamin D supplementation, but there is a definite improvement, more over it helps in development delay, speech improvement so may be very helpful in children with Cerebral palsy with seizures. They also have very limited sunlight exposure.

- Since vitamin D is a harmless vitamin (medication) everybody can start using it before an "RCT" disrupts everything. Even if an RCT proves my assumption equivocal I will be using it for my babies because I am more than convinced.

- Encourage daily sunlight exposure like routine exercise. "Surya-Namaskar" may be a way of getting blessing from sun God.

## Chapter 33

# CLINICALLY NOTED ASSOCIATIONS OF VITAMIN D DEFICIENCY WITH DISEASES AND MECHANISMS OF ACTION OF VITAMIN D

Over the last 100 years human behavior had drastically changed with urbanization and lifestyle changes. Paralleling with that numerous diseases has also crept in silently and we attribute this to our changing food habits, lack of physical activity, stress, excessive intake of environmental toxins through air, water and food. There is increased obesity, diabetes, proliferative diseases, behavioral issues, numerous rare diseases propping up, rare diseases becoming common the list is endless. Even though death from infection has decreased death from other diseases is on the rise. This varied spectrum over the last 100 years can be seen if we take and compare the snapshots of the world from both ends of the century. The pattern of diseases prevalent in developed world, developing world, underdeveloped world is different. As we move up the ladder, we get the new pattern of diseases. The disease pattern from the poorest of African countries may be the disease pattern seen during the beginning of 20$^{th}$ century in North America.

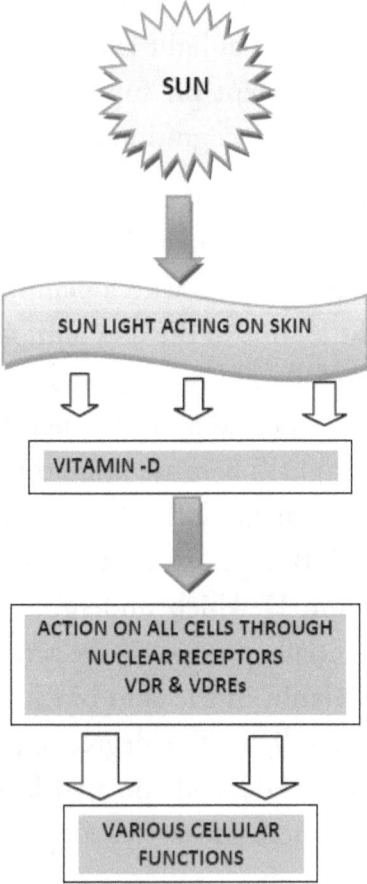

**Figure: 1** Vitamin D production and its action through VDR and VDRE's

I want to bring to the notice a silent human behavioral change happening unknowingly with urbanization. Apart from food habits and decreased physical activity there is increased trend towards apartment culture due to various reasons. Due to apartment culture the chance for sunlight exposure even if you want is reduced dramatically. Virtually mankind is cutoff from sunlight. For travel we use car and whenever we want to walk, we use umbrella for "protection" from sunlight. People are afraid of tanning of skin from sunlight exposure. Virtually we are cutting off from sunlight. What will happen when this essential light is cut off from our life. All the thing the body was dependent on sunlight becomes exposed. But since it is a slow process, its recognition is slow.

Usually most of the food items contains all the nutrients required for us, except vitamin D. Vitamin D from food items is insufficient why is that? Everything God does with a planning and since sunlight is freely available half the time of the day, almighty never expected its deficiency and purposefully did not supplement sufficiently in other food items. God never expected a drastic behavioral change from us of totally avoiding sunlight. There are numerous diseases coming out in the open simply due to the lack of vitamin D deficiency. From sunlight exposure (UVB rays) skin non enzymatically produces inactive form of vitamin D which undergoes hydroxylation in the liver and kidney sequentially producing the active form of vitamin D, i.e., 1,25(OH)2D. Melanin in the skin blocks UVB rays to protect from over exposure to sunlight. The degree of production of vitamin D from sunlight exposure depends on two factors, your skin color (melanin) and the area where you are residing, away from equator the less the intensity of UVB rays.

Active form of vitamin D (1,25(OH)2D) is the ligand for the **Vitamin D Receptor (VDR)**, a transcription factor, binding to the sites in DNA called **Vitamin D Response Elements (VDREs)**. There are thousands of these binding sites regulating hundreds of genes in a cell-specific fashion. VDR-regulated transcription is dependent on co-modulators, the profile of which is also cell specific. Analogs of 1,25(OH)2D are being developed to target specific diseases with minimal side effects. With the finding of vitamin D receptors in nearly every tissue and the more recent discovery of thousands of VDR binding sites throughout the genome controlling hundreds of genes, the interest in vitamin D and its impact on multiple biologic process has accelerated tremendously as evidenced by thousands of publications each year for the past several years. Vitamin D is not like any other vitamins it action is not single pointed like B-complex vitamin or vitamin K or C. It actually helps in the evolution from an embryo to a mature adult. That's why vitamin D deficiency produces severe infertility, cells cannot evolve or cells cannot differentiate into the next stage. Its action is through thousands of genes, comprehension of its action will take decades.

Over my clinical practice I have observed the importance of vitamin D and sunlight exposure and applied this clinically and found good response for my patients. I want to share this information with my fellow doctors. Those who are in institutions can conduct studies for proving or disproving it. The degree of clinical association seen can be grouped into high, moderate and low association.

**Table: 1** Vitamin D deficiency and observed & suspected associations with diseases*

| SI | Observations | Clinical association observed | Comments |
|---|---|---|---|
| 1 | In rickets | High | Also rule out associated hypothyroidism |
| 2 | In delayed eruption of tooth | High | Also rule out associated hypothyroidism |
| 3 | In dental caries and recovery | High | Also rule out associated hypothyroidism |
| 4 | Stunting and growth faltering (Growth failure) | High | Also rule out associated hypothyroidism |
| 5 | Developmental delay | High | Also rule out associated hypothyroidism |
| 6 | Speech delay | High | Also rule out associated hypothyroidism |

| SI | Observations | Clinical association observed | Comments |
|---|---|---|---|
| 7 | Prevention of recurrent febrile seizure | Moderate | |
| 8 | Prevention of recurrent seizure | Moderate | |
| 9 | Prevention of recurrent status epilepticus | Moderate | Rule out channelopathy |
| 10 | Breath holding spells | High | Rule out cardiac causes |
| 11 | In improving immunity | Moderate | Treat primary focus of infection completely and then recurrence decreases |
| 12 | In early stages of autism | High | Good response with vitamin D |
| 13 | In advanced autism | Low | Fixed changes would have occurred |
| 14 | Diabetes control | Moderate | Better diabetic control |
| 15 | Obesity | Moderate / low | Vitamin D requirement doubles or triples |
| 16 | Weakness and lethargy | Moderate | Becomes more energetic |
| 17 | Abnormal / aggressive behavior | Low | Response seen in some patients |
| 18 | Role in re-pigmentation after tinea infection of skin | Moderate | Highly suspicious association of vitamin D deficiency and increased and extensive tinea infection of skin |
| 19 | Vitiligo for re-pigmentation | Moderate | Low vitamin d levels decreases skin pigmentation to increase skin vitamin d production |

| SI | Observations | Clinical association observed | Comments |
|---|---|---|---|
| 20 | Suspected association of low thyroid hormone levels with Vit-D deficiency (↑TSH, ↓FT4) | Doubt full association | High number of borderline cases of hypothyroidism seen associated with vitamin D deficiency |
| 21 | In Anemia | Doubt full association | Anemia invariably accompanies vitamin D deficiency and shows very low response even if iron supplementation are given. |
| 22 | Role in cancer and growth with vit-D deficiency | Good association | Several studies published |
| 23 | Constipation | Doubtful association | Rule out hypothyroidism and subclinical URTI |
| 24 | EEG normalization | Doubtful association, needs studies | Studies can be taken up to see normalization of EEG with vitamin D treatment |
| 25 | In cancer treatment | Moderate | Studies published, several VDRE's developing to specifically target cancer cells. |
| 26 | IUGR babies and low vitamin D in mother | Doubtful | Need research |
| 27 | Low vitamin D levels and high mortality during myocardial infarctions | Moderate | Published papers |
| 28 | Infertility | High | High association with infertility |
| 29 | PIH and preeclampsia | High | Proved through studies |

| SI | Observations | Clinical association observed | Comments |
|---|---|---|---|
| 30 | Vitamin D deficiency and increased covid-19 mortality | ? high association | ??, more death rate seen away from equator and in urban cities and developed countries |
| 31 | In adult osteo-arthritis | Moderate | ? prolonged deficiency |
| 32 | Role in prevention of viral infections | Moderate | Any association of viral epidemic during the winter season with low sunlight exposure. |
| 33 | Death fast approaches once you are bedridden | Low | Is there any role of decreased sunlight exposure and bedridden death |
| 34 | Increased chance for LSCS if you are vitamin D deficient | Low | Studies published; vitamin D deficiency increases your chance for LSCS, muscle function need vitamin D |
| 35 | IUGR and SGA babies | Moderate | Cellular multiplication and differentiation need vitamin D |
| 36 | Inverse relationship with maternal 25(OH) D and amount of tooth decay in infants | High | Proven through studies |
| 37 | Vitamin D deficiency associated with infertility, low birth weight and poor birth outcome | High | Study proven |

\* Some of the observations are from Dr. Micheal F. Holick, a pioneer in vitamin D research

The table-1 shows the associations of vitamin D with various diseases observed, some are already in the open but some are still hiding. Some associations are high and definite improvements seen with interventions. Some are weak associations and all needs definite studies. But studies have its own limitations and individual advantages can disappear in studies, since each case is different this harmless vitamin treatment should not be denied to patients. In several parts of the world vitamin D research is going on in full swing, vitamin D by its action through nuclear receptors have numerous actions through hundreds of genes in most of the tissues, we are still unravelling the mysteries and it will take 5-10 more years to fully dig out all the secrets. It should not be too late for our current babies.

We have to make lifestyle changes of compulsory 15 to 30 minutes sun exposure daily, either as simple open space walk with minimal clothes, or encourage "Surya-namaskar" facing the sun. Ideal time for sunlight exposure is 10 am to 3pm. (UVB rays). Kids should be allowed to play in the open. Fifteen to twenty years ago vitamin D was only considered in the diagnosis of rickets now we have come a long way and we will be travelling a long way forward in future, food fortification of vitamin D is not a distant necessity. Newborn supplementation of vitamin D is a standard protocol now. We are slowly but steadily recognizing the importance of vitamin D. I advise doctors to see some of the lecture videos of Dr. Micheal F. Holick's from internet.

## Chapter 34

# PITFALLS IN SEIZURE MANAGEMENT

Seizure is a very commonly encountered entity in both neonatal and pediatric practice. I am not going into the list of causes or steps in the treatment; I want to discuss some of the pitfalls observed in the management of seizures. We treat most of the referred cases of seizure and had a fairly good success rate. I have some disagreement in principle with some specialist's approach towards seizure management. There are some contentious issues. I call them pit falls in seizure management. Some specialist never aims for full clinical seizure control and some even advised avoiding seizure medications for simple febrile seizures. Simple febrile seizure diagnosis is actually a retrospective diagnosis, full picture is evident only after one or 2 days. Our protocol for seizure includes the following.

1. Aim for complete clinical seizure control.

2. Aim for EEG seizure control.

3. All seizure should be aggressively managed even if that is a simple febrile seizure.

4. Seizures can come in different forms and aim is to control all forms of seizures. Atypical varieties which are continuously present and missed are, constant tonic posturing in a CP child, occasional episodes of posturing, persistent retro colic posturing with increased tone, episodic unprovoked irritability, cry, emotional liability etc. These are due to uncontrolled impulse production from some areas of the brain and spreading. Each episode of seizure has a potential for brain damage.

5. Add anticonvulsants and increase the dose till you get a good response and if not add a second drug. After neonatal period usage of phenobarbitone is less and levetiracetam is a good broad-spectrum drug.

6. Always do Vitamin D estimation whenever child presents with seizures and add vitamin D supplementation in adequate doses.

7. If there are breakthrough seizures even after increasing the dose add a second drug.

8. If clinically seizure free then take an EEG after 3 -4 months and see if EEG has also been normalized. If you are dealing with a developmental delay child improvement is better seen if there is EEG normalization also.

**Table: 1**  Some questions and explanations about seizures

| Statement | Logical explanation |
|---|---|
| Why febrile seizure should always be taken seriously? / why all seizure should be treated aggressively? | When child presents to you, we don't know when the next seizure is and we don't know whether next seizure is a status epilepticus or not. Take all seizures seriously. |
| Why full clinical control of seizure is important? | One basic observation is each episode of seizure produces brain damage and that may not be measurable. Seizure is like arrythmia and over time it produces damage. But we have seen all uncontrolled seizures over time produces regression of mile stones or developmental delay. Missed occasional seizure produces damage to the brain in long run. We trained to detect only tonic clonic seizures, just tonic posturing and other periodic manifestations are missed most of the time. |

| Statement | Logical explanation |
|---|---|
| Why aim for EEG normalization when treating seizure in long term? | Even if there are no clinical seizures, with EEG seizures neurons are in constant uncontrolled firing and so normal developmental sequence and impulse transmission cannot take place and most babies lag in development. Once you normalize EEG you can see better social interactions and developmental processes coming back in babies. |
| Why do vitamin D estimation in all cases of seizures? | We have seen good association with low vitamin D levels and seizures. Recurrence of seizures is very less once vitamin D supplementations are started. |

We aggressively treat seizures either using oral or IV anticonvulsants and don't be hesitant in using multiple anticonvulsants. For me seizure is an uncontrolled firing of impulses from neurons, in the process stimulating any areas of the brain namely motor areas, sensory areas, sub cortical areas producing different clinical manifestations. Any uncontrolled neuronal firing results in ATP deficiency in the cell, damage to organelles and swelling of the neurons, can trigger apoptosis. When seizure is uncontrolled, cerebral oedema ensures, autoregulation gets deranged, respiration becomes compromised, and even result in respiratory failure and death. We have to take any seizure seriously and any recurrent or uncontrolled seizure is a potential candidate for status epilepticus. Seen several cases of seizures, starting as simple febrile seizure and ending in status epilepticus. Seen cases of death where parents took simple febrile seizures callously at home and develop status epilepticus and death on their way to hospital. We give anticonvulsants to all cases of seizure orally or as IV depending on the condition at the time of presentation.

A diagnosis of simple febrile seizure is a retrospective diagnosis and at presentation one can never predict whether a recurrence of seizure will occur or not. Always keep in mind the possibility of recurrence of seizure, which will make you more prepared for a bad eventuality.

**So, avoid seizure pit falls by**

1. Taking all seizures seriously
2. Treating all seizures aggressively
3. All seizures are a potential case for status epilepsy
4. Any seizure is a potential cause for brain damage,
5. Any seizure can turn into a potential life-threatening event (seizure with vomiting and aspiration of gastric contents)
6. Aim for complete clinical seizure control and EEG normalization
7. Vitamin D supplementation after seizure episode can decrease the intensity and frequency of seizures episodes.

## Chapter 35

# A PASSING COMMENT ON NORMAL DISTRIBUTION CURVE (GAUSSIAN DISTRIBUTION)

Everything in this universe has a Gaussian or bell-shaped distribution, may it be weight, height of a human being, blood sugar, cholesterol of a target population, intelligence (IQ) in a population. Details can be read in biostatic books. Whatever value you take the distribution takes the form of a bell shape, with tendency for the values to centralise towards mean and median with values tapering towards periphery. When we derive a normal value for a particular chemical in the body, we take large number of values from a target population thinking that everybody in that group to be normal. Here also you get a bell shaper distribution with tapering of values towards periphery and take central 95 percentile of values {ie, 2-SD (standard deviation)} as normal. There are 2.5 percentile of values outside the 2-SD cut off, majority of these outside values may be abnormal, but normal values may also be there. Similarly, inside 2-SD also there can be abnormal values for that individual but the possibility decreases as we move towards the median values or the $50^{th}$ centile values. For practical purpose we take the central 2 SD values as cuff referral for a population. This is also true for TSH and Free T4 values. When we take this arbitrary 2SD cut off, there are individuals on both sides of the cut of with abnormal values. If we take 4 IU/ml as upper TSH cut off for children, there are children with 4.4 IU/ml TSH with normal thyroid function for that individual (needs no treatment) and there are persons with 3.5 IU/ml TSH value with abnormal thyroid function for that individual (needs treatment). This is because of variations in genetic makeup of individuals, more over there may be several other facilitating factors for thyroid hormones to function which are unknown. If any of these persons show developmental lag then you can be sure that this individual's thyroid value is abnormal and needs external support. That is why we need to give a trial of thyroxine for borderline cases of thyroid values with development lag. General tendency I have observed is to do repeat TSH till you get a normal value and highlight that one and avoid giving treatment to that individual, is this a good strategy? Our strategy should be the reverse of that.

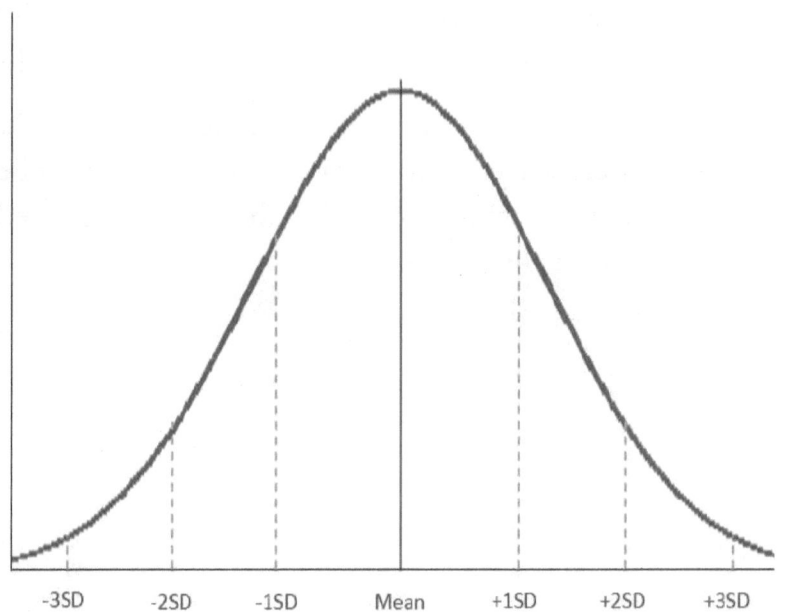

**Figure: 1** Normal distribution curve (Gaussian distribution)

Our problem is oversimplification of human body. It is too complex to be simplified. What is the way out to get out of this trap? The only way is to loosen your grip on the rigid cut offs and values you have artificially made. Moreover, you can see that over the years the TSH cut off has come down from 10 IU/ml. Why is this happening? Because with higher cut off you are not getting the desired results for your patients. That is exactly what is happening for babies with developmental delay with borderline TSH and free T4 values. These borderline cases of hypothyroidism are showing good results on treatment.

We are constantly, but unknowingly using gaussian distribution curve in our day-to-day practice. For example, nurse informed that a patients sodium value is 137 meq/L. our brain immediately analysed it as whether it is nearer to median of the bell-shaped sodium distribution curve or not. The further it is away you are worried. This is the case with all values. Border line values means it is outside 2-SD. Very abnormal value (e.g. Na- 158 meq/L) means it is beyond 3-SD.

So, whenever a borderline value is encountered always take into consideration the clinical condition of the child and then act because the normal cut offs are technical cut offs. There is definite overlap of values near the cut offs in both directions.

## Chapter 36

# PITFALLS LEADING TO BREASTFEEDING FAILURE

No pediatric book is complete without discussing breastfeeding. There are enough books in the shelfs on breastfeeding and so I am not boring you with common discussions on breastfeeding. I will be covering some commonly seen pitfalls leading to breastfeeding failure. Even though we are boasting of high success in breastfeeding the ground reality is not that convincing. Due to simple faults mothers are slowly slipping into top feeding trap, major contributor to this is the health workers. Even though there is high level of training in breastfeeding, when it comes to minute practical aspects there is a deficiency gap. We are having a fairly good success rate in establishing breastfeeding and sustenance. I will just discuss the techniques we use for our successful breastfeeding and also highlight the traps seen on its way.

Gynecologist have a great role to play during antenatal period, by educating mothers about the importance of breastfeeding. They can detect short nipple, retracted nipple, and they can also educate them about the advantages of breastfeeding and make them ready for the task. But don't intervene because of the increased theoretical chance of preterm labor. I wonder anybody of you have ever seen initiation of labor pain with nipple stimulation. I thing that is an extended imagination. The pathway for initiation of labor is not that simple! Doctors can give pamphlets to read, take classes, give links on talks on breastfeeding etc. as part of health education.

Every hospital should have an expert team on breastfeeding who daily visits postnatal mothers and show them exact breastfeeding positions, not theoretical discussions. They also should have a well written policy on the actions to be taken. Points to follow after delivery.

- Immediately after the delivery we can start KMC and breastfeeding on the delivery table itself or start feeding after giving all the primary care the baby needs (cutting of cord, weighing, vitamin K etc.)

- The first staff assisting breastfeeding should take note of any defect in the nipple like short or retracted or large nipple. If any defects are found take corrective steps immediately like for example give syringe correction for retracted nipple. We don't like to find a retracted nipple on the day of discharge. If that happens then it amounts to negligence. Document the findings in the nursing chart, the time of first breastfeeding and comments about the nipple. When they handover to the next duty staff or ward staff hand over the comments about the nipple and the advice given. This proper handover is lacking in most of the institutes, it should not be like every staff discovers the short nipple, once found spread the message. Strict action during this delivery time can prevent several embracing movements later.

- Daily lactation help team should visit postnatal mothers and give advice. They can also visit antenatal mothers.

- Every staff involved should be trained well in breastfeeding.

- Doctors on rounds should ask about the ease of breastfeeding. They should ask 2 questions during rounds.

    - Is there any **nipple pain** – This suggest faulty baby-breast attachment which can result in sore nipples, candid infection of the nipple etc.

- Is there any **breast pain** – It's present suggests engorged breasts (engorged with milk but baby is not feeding because of poor attachment or excessive top feeds) and more frequent breastfeeding is needed and stop top feeds if any is given. Baby is not emptying the breasts properly, so attach the baby to the breast properly, if needed express out the excess milk to make the breasts softer for easy attachment.

- Advise **not to clean the breasts** before each feed (washing with water or by wet wipes). This is done by some sturdy mothers because of fear of infection for their baby. Tell them that no infection spreads from mother to her child, even if that occurs you produces its remedial measures (antibody). The frequent cleaning with wet cloths wipes away the normal protective sebum coating and that can lead to candid infection of the nipple, which causes the nipple to become sore, cracked and painful.

- Be a **"truly baby friendly hospital"**. That means if there is real milk deficiency even after trying all tricks you have to give supervised top feeds with gokarnam or with glass and spoon. Never ask the parents to buy any infant formulae, hospital should provide after instruction from doctors. This is to prevent the misuse later, if you ask to buy parents will continue to use that at home even after good breastmilk output to avoid wasting of milk powder. Tell them about the dangers of bottle feeding. Once breast milk is adequate stop top feed supplementation. **If you 100% strictly follow exclusive breastfeeding (nothing except breastmilk policy) one or two babies in a year end up in serious hypoglycemia and seizures.** Please remember that hypoglycemic seizures have a 50% long term neurologic defects that is a very high percentage and a lifelong burden. Our policy is no hypoglycemic seizure in once life time, that is why I mentioned "truly baby friendly", babies should not starve in your hospital at the same time never over use top feeds. Always label separately the high-risk group for hypoglycemia, they are IUGR babies, <2,5 kg, preterm babies, babies with infection, GDM, LGA babies, mothers with previous feeding problems etc. For all high-risk babies do GRBS estimation for the first 3 days during which most of the transition would have occurred. Don't encourage very early discharges (before 48 hours) before establishing breastfeeding. Your one day saved at hospital can be a long-term curse on you. There should be a definite follow up schedule within a week. This is because most of the problems occur within the first week after discharge – feeding problems, neonatal jaundice, excessive weight loss, hypernatremic dehydration, umbilical sepsis, late onset sepsis etc. No point in scheduling follow-up after 2-3 weeks, either they would have adapted to a new normal, like established top feeds, very high peak of hyperbilirubinemia gone by, very extreme weight loss, presenting with extreme hypernatremic dehydration etc.

- Other faulty tendency seen on follow up are, as soon as the mother say there is no breast milk doctor prescribes top feeds without checking for its truthfulness. Try to find out the cause by asking,
    - How many times baby has passed urine in 24 hours? (>5-6 times is a sign of good milk output)
    - How much time does baby sleeps after feeds? if baby sleeps well after feeds then milk output is likely to be adequate.
    - Is there any weight gain on follow up, if there is weight gain that means there is good milk output? If normal weight loss is seen tell mother that is normal.

- Ask for any pain in the nipple, or breast. Ask your nurses to see the feeding position and note down and correct any faulty techniques.

- Check the feeding position and correct if any faults, ask mother to relax and not to take tension. (pain and stress are the two enemies of successful breastfeeding)

- Painful breast conditions inhibit **prolactin reflex or milk secretion reflex.** Stress, embarrassment, worry and doubt causes suppression of **oxytocin reflex or milk ejection reflex**.

- If there is any defect in technique correct it and ask to come the next week for follow up.

- Practice exclusive breastfeeding till 6 months and advise proper weaning during follow up.

- If there is a real issue of less milk (less milk output is a reality and each mother is different) we can prescribe top milk with the advice to give with Gokarnam or with spoon and instruct specifically not to use bottle. I have seen so many doctors prescribing top feeds and never advising how to feed, tell specifically not to use bottle for feeding. Bottle with nipple is the worst enemy of breastfeeding and not the top milk itself. Ask to give adequate amounts of top feeds 3 to 4 times a day only after sucking at the breast. Don't encourage fixed 2 or 3 hourly top feeds or small quantity frequent feeding just to suppress the crying. These are straight road to breastfeeding failure. As soon as breastmilk output increases you can decrease frequency of top feeds and finally stop it in 1 to 2 weeks' time.

- How to advise mothers who are going to work after 6 months of maternity leave

- Continue breastfeeding whenever mother gets time.

- You can express and keep the breastmilk, use that for next feeding. In room air breastmilk can remain relatively sterile for 4 hours and inside refrigerator for 24 hours. Rewarm the milk by dipping in warm water and never boil breast milk.

- Give top milk 2 to 3 times while at work with Gokarnam or directly with glass. Never using bottle is the secret formula for successfully maintaining breastfeeding while going to work.

- In between you can also give weaning foods 2 to 3 times.

- If your office is nearby, you can come and feed the baby.

- Breastfeed the baby after coming from office and slightly increased night feeding can help you in maintaining milk output. Too much increased night feeding can land up you in trouble latter.

- Mother usually complain of decreased milk output and unsatisfied child after feeding in the latter half of first year and may ask for permission to start top feeds. Tell mother that breastmilk output flattens after 6 months of age and now their babies need more weaning foods to sustain growth. If you give more milk or other liquid diets their babies weight will only flattened out.

- Whenever your patient is a healthcare worker (doctors or nursing staff) I tell my team to be doubly vigilant and treat them as high-risk group. The reasons are many, they are highly resistant to suggestions, some already have some wrong notions that we we have to remove first, then only they will take new suggestions. You have to practically show them the position because they will invariably say they know everything. I tell the sisters to put double the effort towards health care workers. Only a rare minority of health care workers, who had worked in a good institution with good maternal and child care setup knows exactly what to do, so for practical purpose you can ignore this group.

- There is a tendency for mothers to keep up the same frequency of breastfeeding and continue to give 8 to 10 times breastmilk. There is no time for any other feeds and babies weight gaining stops. There is also a tendency to increase night feeding frequency which is bad for the baby in the long run. In India most children's weight get stuck in the range of 7.5kg and 9kg till they are relieved from breastfeeding. This is due to the milk addiction and excessive night time feeding. Less solid food enters the child and child is addicted to breastmilk and child also becomes more irritable and anemic and never leaves the mothers surroundings.

- Why is the problem with excessive night time feeding? Excessive night feeding causes baby to take less food in the day time. This is because GIT needs some rest in 24 hours and it takes rest during day time by decreasing appetite and slowing digestion.

- Advise mother to decrease breastmilk feeding frequency as child matures and stop feeding by 2 years of age.

- Is extending breastfeeding beyond 1.5 years of age has any advantages? Is there a relationship between excessive breastfeeding during the 1.5 years to 2 years age group and stunting in children? This is a debatable topic. There is a growth flattening happening in children who are depending on excessive breastmilk feeding beyond 1 years of age, especially those addicted to nigh time feeding. This is only my observation, have you observed this. How many percentages of children in western countries continue breastfeeding beyond 1 year of age? The American academy of Pediatrics (AAP) recommends breastfeeding for the first 12 months of age and "thereafter for as long as mother and baby desire". WHO recommends the practice up to age 2 "or beyond".

## Chapter 37

# HOW TO PREVENT ANTIBIOTIC MISUSES IN OUR COUNTRY?

Antibiotics are the only weapon available against microorganisms and that arsenal is fast depleting and our enemy is acquiring new and new weapons and, in the meantime, we are misusing whatever is available with us. One thing is clear we cannot permanently dominate the microorganism forever, that is an impossible dream. But we can use our weapons tactically to our advantage. First and foremost, in any battle is "know your enemy before the battle". Most of the time we are blindly into the battle without knowing our enemy (not knowing the kind of organisms) and using useless weapons endlessly. Antibiotic resistance is rampant in our community and not to mention in the hospital. In hospital it is a playground for MDR and PDR organisms. The following are my observations for the development of antibiotic resistance menace in our country and ways to avoiding it.

1. Stop availability of "cheap" and subquality drugs, antibiotics should have strict quality control and price should not be a criterion for that. Cheap drug should never be subquality drug. Prices goes up once quality control kicks in. Our national quality control bar should be comparable with that of western countries and it should not be lowered.

2. Three-day course of antibiotic prescriptions should be banned, it should be 5 to 10 to 14 days course. Most of the time when fever subsides antibiotic is stopped but full cure of infection is still doubtful. The remaining organism is the

one which survived the antibiotic on slot and these are the once which will multiply later, the antibiotic resistant brood.

3. Never to dispense antibiotic without a fresh prescription, put heavy penalty on the law breakers.

4. Chemist should always dispense full course of antibiotic, that is if 2 bottles are required then they should not dispense one bottle.

5. Make available 60 ml or 100 ml bottles for antibiotics. There is a resistance to buy 2 bottles of antibiotic, they buy one bottle and stop antibiotics once fever and other major symptoms subsides.

6. Underdosing is a problem in pediatrics (vomiting and resistance to take medications), so, from our part never write under dosage for our kids. Underdosage of substandard drugs for inadequate duration will create a menace.

7. Doctors should also do culture and sensitivity to find the organism they are dealing with. Policy should be to know the enemy. Always do a throat swab culture and sensitivity for upper respiratory tract infections, mostly the same organisms spreads in the family. Know your enemy well.

8. Accept the reality that amoxicillin and ampicillin are > 80% resistant in the community. These cannot cure all your infections.

9. Identify chronic carriers and chronic spreaders in the community and treat them completely even if that require IV antibiotics.

10. Super spreaders should never be labelled "allergic", they may hide behind this label and escape detection and they continuously spread in the community. Do throat and

nostril swab for culture and sensitivity, don't be surprised to find a MRSA or a PDR / MDR gram negative organisms.

11. If you find a chronic infection in a family try to find its source which can be a well water contamination from as septic tank, or a chronic carrier in the family.

12. More than 90% of infection coming to our OPD are URTI and so make throat examination a habit and throat C&S a routine when ever there is resistance towards complete cure. Don't aim for symptomatic cure.

13. Ban all higher antibiotic use in cattle and poultry industry and should be used only under higher level supervision. The rampant use has caused resistance towards polymyxin and fluroquinolones in the community.

14. Daily sunlight exposure to all individuals should be a trend like daily exercise and vitamin D has a huge role to play in immunity. Encourage daily sunlight exposure like daily exercise, so do daily outdoor exercises.

The moment you are born your surrounding organisms try to colonize you and it's a constant fight between them and you. This will continue till your death and mostly these commensals will be your cause of death if your death happens to be sepsis related. Colonization with organism which you cannot avoid, it is better to colonize with a less aggressive organism. But during your course of life, you will definitely get colonized with more aggressive organisms depending on the organisms you are exposed. Only escape is to ramp up your immunity and take complete cure from any infections and never act as a carrier of resistant organisms.

During these years of my practice, I have seen several doctors prescribing the same antibiotics several times even if their patient is not completely recovering. An antibiotic if it is not curing an infection even after 5 days it is unlikely to cure the infection even if used for 10 or 14 days. You are dealing with a resistant organism. Do a culture and change to another category of antibiotics.

## Chapter 38

# WHOLE-BODY COOLING IN RESISTANT NEONATAL SEIZURES AS A NEURO PROTECTIVE STRATEGY.

It is proven beyond doubt that whole body cooling has a neuroprotective effect in Hypoxic Ischemic Encephalopathy (HIE). Why can't we use that same neuroprotective strategy in babies with uncontrolled neonatal seizures. In our NICU we have used this for 5 to 6 babies with good success.

Seizure in a baby if recurrent or continuous is going to damage the brain. Seizure produces continuous firing from the cells beyond its capacity and it exhausts all its energy reserves and its basic metabolism suffers and if prolonged it can result in cytotoxic cell death or apoptosis. Babies can come with different types of presentations like continuous seizure outside your hospital and then referred to you or there can be continuous seizure for a baby already in your NICU. If seizure can be controlled with one or two medication quickly no need for whole body cooling. But referred outside newborns can have prolonged seizures either unrecognized or not properly treated.

If the baby is having shock and sepsis correct it quickly and then you can start cooling the baby. Once baby is cooled seizure subsides very fast. Give the usual choices of anticonvulsants. You are cooling for neuroprotection from seizures. In NICU all kinds of seizures are not damaging to the brain but some are definitely like for example hypoglycemic seizures and HIE related seizures. Needs good study for seeing the effects of neuroprotection in hypoglycemic seizures as it is proven that 50% of babies with hypoglycemic seizures will have neurodevelopmental abnormalities.

Cooling is done as usual for the HIE babies, we use coolant pack and air conditioning system. We do cooling for 1 to 3 days depending on the severity of insult and fastness of recovery. All our babies had an excellent recovery and long-term outcome. Since cooling technique is an already proven method of neuroprotection, this can be utilized for neuroprotection in other diseases also. I wonder why this hesitancy for using in other diseases. Other NICUs can take up this and apply to their babies. Failure of cooling mostly occurs when the shock and sepsis are uncontrollable.

# REFERENCES

1. Nelson textbook of pediatrics 21st edition
2. Neurology of the newborn, Joseph J Volpe 5th edition
3. Manual of neonatal care, John P. Cloherty 8th edition
4. BLS, Basic Life Support, Provider manual, 2015, American heart Association
5. PALS, Pediatric Advance Life support, ACLS Provider manual 2015.
6. NALS, Textbook of Neonatal Resuscitation, 7th Ed.
7. The Royal Children's Hospital Melbourne guidelines on Vitamin D recommendation, endorsed by Paediatric improvement Collaborative. 2020 update
8. Peter S. Aronson, Gerhard Giebisch, "Effect of pH on Potassium: New Explanations for Old Observations" J Am Soc nephrol. 2011 Nov; 22(11): 1981-1989.doi: 10.1681/ASN.2011040414 PMCID: PMC3231780 PMID: 21980112.
9. Flemming Cornelius, Naoki Tsunekawa, Chikashi Toyoshima, Disctinct pH dependencies of Na+/K+ selectivity at the two faces of Na,K-ATPase, Journal of Biological Chemistry, doi: https://doi.org/10.1074/jbc.RA117.000700
10. T. Rajini Samuel, Kolanati Prudhvi, Pulluru Nithin Kumar, Nurukurti Surya Sravani et al. Assessment of ionized calcium levels in various acid base disorders in ICU patients, Int. J. Pharm. Sci. rev. Res., 49(1), March-April 2008, Article No. 10, pages:60-64

11. Biondi B. the Normal TSH Reference Range: What Has Changed in the Last Decade? J Clin Endocrinol meta. 2013: 98(9): 3584-3587. Doi: 10.1210/jc.2013-2760. [PubMed] [CrossRef] [Google Scolar]

12. Thyroid Hormones in Brain Development and Function, Bernal J, ncbi.nlm.nih.gov

13. Krzysztof Lewandowski, Reference range of TSH and Thyroid Hormones, Thyroid Res. 2015; 8(suppl 1): A17. Published online 2015 jun 22 doi: 10.1186/1756-6614-8-S1-A17. PMCID: PMC4480274.

14. Christopher N Andrews, Martin Storr, Pathophysiology of chronic constipation Can J Gastroenterol. 2011 Oct; 25 (Suppl B): 16B-21B.

15. Gillessen T Budd SL, Lipton SA, Excitatory Amino Acid Neurotoxicity. Ncbi.nlm.nih.gov

16. Kelly, AM, McAlpine, R, Kyle, E. venous pH can safely replace arterial pH in the initial evaluation of patients in the emergency department. Emerg med J. 2001: 18:340-342

17. Usher R, Reduction of mortality from respiratory distress syndrome of prematurity with early administration of intravenous glucose and sodium bicarbonate. Paediatrics 1963; 32 (6): 966-75

18. Afrin M, role of Sodium Bicarbonate to treat Neonatal Metabolic Acidosis: Beneficial or Not. J Bangladesh Coll Phys Surg 2017: 35: 80-85

19. Forsythe SM, Schmidt GA, sodium bicarbonate for the treatment of lactic acidosis. Chest 2000; 117:260-67

20. Shapiro J L, Functional and metabolic response of isolated heart to acidosis: effects of sodium bicarbonate and carbicarb. Am J Physiol 1990; 258:H1835-H1839

21. Kelly, AM. Can VBG analysis replace ABG analysis in emergency care? Emerg Med J. 2016: 33: 152-153.

22. Flemming C, Naoki T, Chikashi T. Distinct pH dependencies of Na+/K+ - selectivity at the two faces of Na K –ATPase. journal of Biological Chemistry, 2018, 293: 2195-2205.

23. Petrus S S, Svetlana N K, Lilia V T, Wolfgang S, Larisa Vasilets. Extracellular pH modulates kinetics of Na K –ATPase. Biochimica et Biophysica Acta 1509 (2000) 496-504

24. Salonikidis, P. S., Kirichenko, S. N., Tajanenko, L.V., Schwarz, W., and Vasilets, L. A. (2000). Extracellular pH modulates kinetics of the Na+,K+-ATPase. Biochim. Biophys. Acta 1509, 496-

25. Kaplan, J. H. (2002). Biochemistry of Na,K-ATPase. Annu. Rev. Biochem. 71:511-535.

www.ingramcontent.com/pod-product-compliance
Lightning Source LLC
Chambersburg PA
CBHW020854180526
45163CB00007B/2502